PROFILES OF THE NUTRIENTS

3. WATER-SOLUBLE AND FAT-SOLUBLE VITAMINS

PROFILES OF THE NUTRIENTS

3. Water-Soluble and Fat-Soluble Vitamins

RICHARD RYDON

Non-fiction

First Paperback Edition: December 2016

ISBN: 978-1-326-80647-7

Cover image – ID 7499030 – tonobalaguer/123RF.com

CONTENTS

Preface

46. Introduction to the Vitamins
47. Vitamin C
48. Choline
49. Niacin
50. Pantothenic Acid
51. Vitamin B_6
52. Riboflavin
53. Thiamine
54. Folate
55. Biotin
56. Vitamin B_{12}
57. Vitamin E
58. Vitamin A (and the Carotenoids)
59. Vitamin K (and Coenzyme Q_{10})
60. Vitamin D
61. Are There Other Vitamins?
62. Some Links Between Nutrients
63. Some Nonvitamins
    Bioflavonoids, Carnitine, Phospholipid Factors, *para-*Aminobenzoic Acid, Taurine, Nucleic Acid Factors, Lipoic Acid, Pangamic Acid and Laetrile.
64. Trace Poisons
65. Dried Products, Herbs and Spices

A5. Loss of Vitamins
A6. Experimental Depletion of Vitamins
A7. Generic Descriptors for Vitamin Activity and Vitamers
A8. Vitamins as Coenzymes
A9 New Units for Older Vitamin Units
A10. Common Toxicity and Deficiency Symptoms of Vitamins

Bibliography
About the Author

Preface

This series of three books includes an account of the nutrients known to be essential for human life. Appropriately, the text is called PROFILES OF THE NUTRIENTS. The series covers some fifty different nutrients. It is intended primarily as an outline for those who seek an introduction to the nutrients presented in a direct way.

The classical definition of a nutrient is an essential substance in food that provides structural or functional components or energy to the body. The ability to provide energy requires one other essential substance that does not come from food, namely oxygen gas.

There are no value judgements on the special merits of selected nutrients. All are equally essential for human life. Each nutrient is identified in the text by:

- A Chapter of its own
- Common name and alternative names
- Some key historical dates (e.g. for the discovery of the vitamins)
- The Nature of each nutrient
- Biological functions
- Daily requirement and food sources
- Toxicity symptoms
- Deficiency symptoms

Book 1 considers carbohydrate, lipid and protein, book 2 considers minerals and trace elements and book 3 considers vitamins. Overall, the series presents a concise outline of each of the essential nutrients.

46

Introduction to the Vitamins

Vitamins are independent organic substances occurring in natural foods in variable amounts either as such or as utilisable precursors which are required in minute amounts for normal health and efficiency.

Vitamins participate in the essential bodily processes of growth, maintenance and reproduction. They are completely independent of one another and distinct from carbohydrates, lipids, proteins, nucleic acids or their simpler components. Hence they exclude, by definition, certain essential fatty acids and amino acids. They do not undergo metabolism for the purposes of providing energy, nor do they serve as components of the major structures in the body. Vitamins are not normally formed in adequate amounts, if at all, in the body tissues. However, sometimes vitamins are provided by the gut flora (bacteria) and hence may not be required specifically in the diet.

The biochemical role of vitamins is largely catalytic. All the B-group vitamins, for example, are known to form parts of the structures (called coenzymes) of various enzymes. When the body is severely deficient in any vitamin, specific clinical diseases may develop because of the breakdown of vital metabolic processes in the cell. These diseases can only be cured by supplying the associated indispensable vitamin and not any other. Persistent inadequate intake of vitamins generally leads to states of lowered biochemical, physiological and even mental well-being. However, in general, the precise connections between the biological role of the vitamins and the clinically observed manifestations of deficiency are not all fully understood.

The total number of known vitamins, recognised to be essential for human life, is fourteen; ten water-soluble and four fat-soluble vitamins. Of the water-soluble vitamins, one is called vitamin C and the other nine are called B-group vitamins. These are listed in Tables 46.1 and 46.2. For convenience, vitamin C will be considered first, then the B-group vitamins and, lastly, the fat-soluble vitamins E, A, K and D, in that order.

A number of substances, called vitamers, may have the same biological activity but in varying degrees. If such substances occur naturally they are considered to form part of a single group, and are usually given a convenient generic designation, such as vitamin D which is in fact several different, although closely related, substances (see Appendix A7). A vitamer is any one of several related chemical compounds that fulfill the same specific vitamin function. The vitamin activity of multiple vitamers is due to the body's ability to convert one vitamer to another or to an active form. Typically, not all vitamers possess exactly the same vitamin potency. This is due to differences in absorption and interconversion of the various vitamers. Often, for the same reason, the toxicity of vitamers can vary. The vitamins themselves vary in their stability during food processing, storage and cooking. Further details on vitamin losses are summarised in Appendix A5.

It can be seen, from the above discussion, that a rigorous definition of the term vitamin is a fairly complex one.

It should be noted that several factors determine the individual requirement for each vitamin. These include the usual variables of age, sex and sometimes activity. In addition, there may be an increased need for certain vitamins during and immediately after various illnesses. During fevers for example the rate of destruction of the vitamins in the body is increased. An excess of certain vitamins may precipitate a deficiency of others. This is particularly true for members of the vitamin B group, and should act as a warning against overdosing.

The daily vitamin requirement is an approximate figure. The gut bacteria supply part of the daily requirement for several vitamins and probably most, of the requirement for biotin and vitamin K.

Therefore, during certain antibiotic therapies, if the gut bacteria have been depleted, there may be an increased need for increased dietary sources of certain vitamins. Vitamin D cannot be produced in the body except by the action of sunlight on the skin. In winter months, there may be an increased need for pre-formed vitamin D in the diet. The niacin requirement varies inversely according to the amount of tryptophan in the diet. In fact, the daily requirement for niacin can be completely replaced if there is sufficient tryptophan in the diet. Several vitamins, particularly vitamins C, B_{12} and A, can be stored in the body hence a deficient intake over several months, even years in some cases, may not produce any symptoms. Of all fourteen vitamins, only four may, under certain circumstances, be adequately supplied with minimal help of dietary sources. These four namely, choline, niacin, biotin and vitamin K, may be termed conditionally essential to distinguish them from nutrients that are absolutely essential and which must be predominantly if not completely supplied in the diet.

In addition to the true vitamins, there are a number of nonvitamins with sufficient biological activity to warrant their special consideration. Some of these are synthesised in adequate amounts in the body from other substances. Others are of therapeutic importance and frequently accompany the true vitamins in nature. These are not considered to be nutritionally essential. Table 46.3 lists a number of these nonvitamins, which will be considered in a separate chapter (Chapter 63).

Some of the vitamin names are generic names which include a number of compounds categorised by a particular activity. See also Appendix A7. A summary of the effects of an excess and a lack of the vitamins, is given in Appendix A10. In the following chapters, details on the history, nature, function, requirement and distribution, toxicity and deficiency of each vitamin will be considered.

Table 46.1. Vitamins stored in the adult human body

VITAMIN	APPROXIMATE AMOUNT (milligrams)
Vitamin E	4,000
Vitamin C	2,500
Niacin	2,000
Pantothenic acid	700
Choline	600
Vitamin A	500
Riboflavin	150
Vitamin B_6	120
Thiamine	70
Vitamin K	30
Folate	15
Vitamin D	10
Biotin	7
Vitamin B_{12}	3

All the above values are highly variable and depend on body weight and nutritional status.

Table 46.2. Relative adult requirement of the vitamins (all values in micrograms per day)

VITAMIN	MALES	FEMALES
Water-soluble		
Vitamin C	90,000	75,000
B-Group Vitamins		
Choline	550,000	425,000
Niacin	16,000	14,000
Pantothenic acid	5,000	5,000
Vitamin B_6	1,700	1,500
Riboflavin	1,300	1,100
Thiamine	1,200	1,100
Folate	400	400
Biotin	30	30
Vitamin B_{12}	2.4	2.4
Fat-soluble		
Vitamin E	15,000	15,000
Vitamin A	900	700
Vitamin K	120	90
Vitamin D	15	15

Table 46.3. Some nonvitamins.

NAME	OCCURENCE

Bioflavonoids
Factors associated with Vitamin C.

L-Carnitine
Factor associated with the B-group vitamins and involved in lipid metabolism.

Choline *, *myo*-Inositol
Factors which are part of certain phospholipids such as Lecithin. Generally considered part of the vitamin B group.

para-Aminobenzoic acid (PABA)
A non-α–amino acid factor which is part of folic acid, and is sometimes termed 'a vitamin within a vitamin'.

Taurine
Another non-α–amino acid factor.

Adenine, Adenylic acid, Orotic acid
Factors which are associated with nucleic acid metabolism. Once considered part of the vitamin B group.

Lipoic acid
A fat-soluble factor not related to other fat-soluble vitamins, but with some structural similarities to biotin. Involved in lipid metabolism.

Pangamic acid, Laetrile (Amygdalin)
Factors associated with the vitamin B group and in particular the apricot kernel.

---

* Choline has been recently classified as a vitamin.

In the context used here, a nonvitamin is a natural substance with certain vitamin-like properties but is not an essential nutrient. The bioflavonoids comprise a wide group of related substances of plant origin.

47

Vitamin C

Common names

Vitamin C.
Ascorbic Acid.

Alternative names

L-Ascorbic acid. Dehydroascorbic acid. Ascorbyl moiety.
Hexuronic Acid. L-Xyloascorbic acid. Cevitaminic acid. Anti-skorbutin. Antiscorbutic factor. Antiscorbutic vitamin. Anti-scurry vitamin. Antioxidant vitamin. Fresh fruit vitamin.

Some of the above terms are archaic and no longer in use. Some terms are trivial.

History

-----: Scurvy has been known for centuries.

circa 1535: Newfoundland Indians first tell mariners how to cure scurvy.

1570: Lancaster prevented scurry by giving crews lemon juice daily.

1757: Lind stated that fresh fruit and vegetables alone protect against scurvy.

1804: The British Navy orders lemon juice rations for all crews.

1907: Holst and Frøhlich produced scurvy in guinea-pigs.

circa 1918: Zilva, *et al.* describe a factor which they isolated from lemon juice. The factor is oxidised by air and is required for development of teeth in animals. Later they show it to be an antiscorbutic agent.

1920: Drummond names the anti-scurvy factor vitamin C. In the same year, he proposes that the final 'e' of the term vitamine be dropped because not all vitamins are amines.

1930: McKinnis and King suggest that vitamin C has reducing properties.

1932: Vitamin C was first isolated from cayenne pepper by Szent-Györgyi, who also isolated it from orange juice, cabbage, and the adrenal cortex. Concurrently, the same hexuronic acid was isolated and crystallised by King and Waugh and recognised as the antiscorbutic agent.

1933: Haworth establishes the structure of hexuronic acid. Reichstein produces synthetic Vitamin C for the first time. Haworth and Szent-Györgyi re-name hexuronic acid as ascorbic acid.

-----: Vitamin C is now a generic term for all compounds that exhibit qualitatively the biological activity of ascorbic acid.

Nature

Vitamin C is structurally related to the carbohydrates, having 6 carbon atoms and several hydroxyl groups. In fact, it is derived from glucose in four steps, the last of which is missing in humans, to yield L-ascorbic acid. Ascorbic acid is an essential vitamin in only a few species of animals. The vitamin is synthesised by most higher plants, microorganisms and animals. The few exceptions include the primates, for example monkeys and humans, the guinea pig, and some rare birds such as the red-vented bulbul bird and the Indian fruit eating bat.

The term vitamin C is now strictly used as a generic descriptor for all substances with ascorbic acid activity. Ascorbic acid itself is taken as the most representative compound of the vitamin C group. It is also the only substance (together with its equally active dehydro- form), which is of natural importance. In other words, ascorbic acid and vitamin C can be taken as virtually synonymous. Vitamin C is not available from the gut bacteria in humans. A large number of synthetic derivatives of ascorbic acid have been studied in recent years but none are more active than the natural compound. The potencies of a number of these compounds are illustrated in Table 47.1. Ascorbic acid is reversibly oxidised to dehydroascorbic acid. Both forms are equally active and occur in the body, with 95 to 90 percent as ascorbic acid and 5 to 10 percent as dehydroascorbic acid. Only the L-isomer is biologically active. The D-isomer has no activity. Vitamin C is a very unstable vitamin. It has been observed that some Indian women during lactation lose more vitamin C in their milk and their urine than they gain in their diet. Perhaps humans, under certain rare conditions, can synthesise some vitamin C.

Biological Functions

- Antioxidants, like ascorbic acid, are reducing agents that neutralise free radicals and protect the cell from damage. As redox catalysts, they can neutralize reactive oxygen species such as hydrogen peroxide. Vitamin C acts as a powerful reducing agent, in which capacity it may protect certain enzymes from oxidation. However, no biological oxidation system has yet been discovered in which ascorbic acid or any of its derivatives serves as a specific coenzyme. For convenience, Appendix A8 lists the coenzyme forms of various vitamins. Ascorbic acid can reduce methaemoglobin, a derivative of the oxygen carrying protein myoglobin found in muscle. It can also reduce some cytochromes, the hydrogen and electron transport carriers found in all cells.

- Vitamin C also helps to counteract toxins, and can prevent oxidative damage caused by heavy metals and promotes the elimination of certain heavy metals from the body, including lead, mercury and copper.

- Vitamin C is essential for the hydroxylation of proline in the synthesis of hydroxyproline. It is also involved in the hydroxylation of lysine to hydroxylysine. Hydroxyproline and hydroxylysine are essential components of collagen, the structural protein of connective tissue, cartilage and capillaries. Collagen is also found in bone. Hence vitamin C is essential for the health of bone, teeth and gums, and the healing of wounds and fractures. The importance of vitamin C is highlighted when it is considered that 30 percent of the total bone protein is in the form of collagen.

- Vitamin C enhances iron absorption from the gut. It acts by converting ferric to ferrous iron, which is more readily absorbed. It also helps to mobilise iron from the ferritin stores in the body.

- Vitamin C is involved in protecting the body against stress. The human body as a whole can store up to 5 grams of ascorbic acid when fully saturated. Much of the vitamin is concentrated in the extracellular fluids, the white blood cells and in the adrenal cortex. Some is also found in the pituitary gland in the brain. The vitamin C in the adrenal cortex is rapidly depleted when the gland is stimulated by adrenocorticotrophic hormone (ACTH) which is released by the pituitary gland. The hormone ACTH, working together with vitamin C stimulates the production on the anti-stress hormones called corticosteroids, in the adrenal cortex itself. Vitamin C is also rapidly depleted following stress, various infections, and fevers in the body. Hence, it has been postulated that the vitamin acts to protect the body in these situations.

- Vitamin C may be involved in the metabolism of the amino acid tyrosine in the body. Tyrosine is converted into *p*-hydroxyphenylpyruvic acid, and this may be further converted into homogentisic acid. Similarly, tryptamine is converted into serotonin (5-hydroxytryptamine). Vitamin C is also involved in the synthesis of noradrenaline. The latter substances are important brain and nerve substances, respectively.

- It can be seen that ascorbic acid, often in association with iron, is involved in a number of hydroxylation reactions in the body, although in some cases these reactions can proceed in the absence of the vitamin. Another such reaction is the conversion of γ–butyrobetaine to carnitine, which is involved in lipid metabolism.

- The dehydroascorbic acid form of the vitamin may be reduced by glutathione in the body. Glutathione itself is an important protective compound particularly with regard to enzymes.

- An oxidised form of the vitamin, possibly monodehydroascorbic acid, may be involved, together with the enzyme ascorbate reductase and sulfhydryl groups (–SH), in the reoxidation of reduced forms of the niacin coenzymes, NADH and NADP. See also Chapter 49.

- Vitamin C may be involved in activating folate in some animals but this role in humans is not yet established.

- Vitamin C may be involved in lipid metabolism and helps maintain low levels of cholesterol in the blood.

- Vitamin C is involved in maintaining the immune system in good condition. Also, high doses of vitamin C are believed to inhibit the replication of certain viruses and bacteria.

- Vitamin C may also counteract some of the effects of histamine in the body and therefore act as an anti-allergic factor. The above findings may form the basis of the widely held, but as yet unproven, hypothesis that vitamin C can prevent the common cold, or at least ameliorate some of its symptoms.

- Vitamin C may inhibit the formation of nitrosamines from nitrates and nitrites, which are used as food preservatives. Nitrosamines are believed to be one cause of cancer.

- Vitamin C may help certain animals to withstand the effects of low temperatures. The significance of this effect is unknown.

- It has been claimed that the reduced form of vitamin C may decrease the requirement for several other vitamins in certain experimental animals. Among the vitamins spared are pantothenic acid, riboflavin, thiamine, folate, vitamin E and vitamin A. Again, the significance of these observations in the human, if any, is as yet unknown.

Requirement

The daily intake of vitamin C is generally around 100 mg per day in well balanced Western diets. The best sources of the vitamin are fresh vegetables and fruit. Some 50 percent of our daily requirement is provided by vegetables and a further 40 percent comes from fruit. The suggested adult intakes of vitamin C are around 90 mg per day for males and 75 mg per day for females, respectively. Higher intakes are required for pregnant and especially lactating females. Intakes of at least 100 mg per day are generally advisable for regular smokers. A vitamin C compendium is included for reference (Table 47.2).

Considerable controversy (more than for any other nutrient), surrounds the setting of the daily allowances for vitamin C. Values have been suggested from as little as 10 mg per day to several thousand times that amount! The absolute minimum daily amount required by adults to prevent scurvy seems to be about 5 mg, and about 10 mg per day will cure scurvy once it has developed. However more than this is necessary for optimum health. Various World authorities have recommended daily intakes ranging from 30 to 100 mg. However, during infections, injury, stress, drug therapies, and many disturbances of health including smoking and heavy drinking, optimum intakes of the vitamin have been estimated at times to be as high as 500 to 1,000 mg for children and 1,000 to 4,000 mg for adults. Some authors even recommend higher values approaching 9 grams per day for adults, but such values seem to have little foundation in practice even though they are generally without toxic side effects.

In extreme cases, doses from 25 to 90 grams of sodium ascorbate have been administered (intravenously) to chronically ill patients such as cancer patients and drug addicts, in an attempt to ameliorate their symptoms. The fact that the body tissues become saturated with intakes of about 200 mg vitamin C per day would seem to indicate that higher intakes are in most cases non-productive. Many authors even argue that general good health is achieved at less than full body saturation with vitamin C.

Toxicity

Excess vitamin C is either metabolised or rapidly eliminated in the urine. Consequently, high doses of vitamin C are relatively non-toxic although several side effects of very high intakes have been reported. Mild nausea, diarrhoea and stomach cramps occur occasionally with doses as low as a few grams per day. The laxative effect is seen by some as a beneficial effect. At one stage, it was thought that high levels of ascorbic acid may metabolise to enough oxalic acid to cause kidney stones. While it is true that high vitamin C intake promotes the excretion of oxalic acid in the urine, this is mostly due to its mild diuretic effect. However, very high intakes of vitamin C can cause an oxalate nephrotoxicity. Vitamin C may also promote the excretion of uric acid, another insoluble compound. Very high intakes may also cause depletion of certain minerals such as copper. High doses of vitamin C can interfere with some anticoagulant drugs used to prevent blood clots in certain patients. Very rarely, skin rashes have occurred in people on high doses of vitamin C. Finally, there may be a rebound effect resulting in some mild scurvy-like symptoms if persons on high doses of vitamin C suddenly stop taking supplements. This may have to do with the body adjusting from a chronically high level of the vitamin to a sudden low level status. But the effect has not been reported very often, and does not seen to occur in experimental animals. Some clinical tests may give false results in patients who are taking high levels of vitamin C. Ascorbic acid excreted in urine can also undergo a chemical conversion to oxalic acid unless a preservative is added to the urine sample.

Deficiency

Smoking depletes vitamin C in the body. Heavy drinking also causes the rapid elimination of vitamin C from the body. Unfortunately, the two habits often go together to compound the problem. Vitamin C is also depleted following the use of many drugs, including aspirin, pain killers, the contraceptive pill, and many antibiotics and sleeping pills. In this regard, it is not clear if older people require additional vitamin C, but many such people are on some form of medication and unfortunately some do not always eat a balanced diet containing fresh vegetables or fruit. All forms of stress (even the competitive physical hardships endured by a trained athlete) tend to deplete the body stores of vitamin C. When fully saturated, the human body can contain up to

5 grams of vitamin C, but this can only be achieved on intakes of 200 mg per day. Intakes of around 45 mg per day maintain the body pool of vitamin C at around 1.5 grams This is generally considered adequate for most healthy individuals. The blood plasma level of ascorbic acid in healthy individuals ranges from about 5 to 15 mg per litre. The value in blood platelets varies from 30 to 75 μg per 10^{10} platelets. And the value in the white blood cell is normally around 160 μg per litre of white cells.

Human ascorbic acid deficiency has been studied in detail under controlled conditions. Within 20 days both the plasma level and the concentration in white cells falls by over 90 percent. After about 120 days, enlarged hair follicles appear which become keratotic. After about 150 days these follicles become haemorrhagic and may be affected all over the body. And after 180 days the severest symptoms of scurvy develop, such as sore bleeding gums, loose teeth, extensive haemorrhages, nose-bleeds and bruising under the skin, falling hair, oedema, anaemia, pains in the joints, loss of appetite, impaired healing of wounds and fractures and even breakdown of old wound tissue and scars. There is also an overall lowered resistance to infection. The walls of the small capillaries breakdown, resulting in tiny blood clots which in extreme cases may accumulate to cause strokes or heart attacks. A consequence of the anaemia is a shortage of breath. In women, poor lactation may result. In children, there is a weakened formation of enamel or dentine of teeth and poor bone growth. Scurry causes an overall weakness and apathy. Fortunately, most of these symptoms can be reversed quickly by supplementation with vitamin C. An improvement may be noticed within a few days, but treatment should continue for several weeks for full recovery. Onset times for various vitamin deficiencies are listed in Appendix A6. Also for convenience, terms now used as generic descriptors for various compounds with related vitamin activities are listed in Appendix A7.

Table 47.1. Relative biopotency of different forms of Vitamin C

NAME	NOMINAL VALUE (percent)
Natural Forms	
L-Ascorbic acid	100
Dehydro-L-ascorbic acid	100
Sodium ascorbate	88
Calcium ascorbate dihydrate	82
Ascorbyl palmitate	42
Synthetic Forms	
6-Deoxy-L-ascorbic acid	30
D-Araboascorbic acid	4
3-O-Methylether derivative	3
Heptono-L-ascorbic acid	1
D-Ascorbic acid	0
Diketogulonic acid	0

The synthetic forms are not used, as L-ascorbic acid itself is readily available as a supplement. Diketogulonic acid is an inactive breakdown product of vitamin C in the body.

Table 47.2. Vitamin C compendium

FOOD GROUP	VITAMIN C LEVEL
Milk and products	Nil
Eggs	Nil
Meat and fish	Nil, variable
Fats and oils	Nil
Grain and products	Nil
Nuts and pulses	Nil
Root vegetables	High
Leaf vegetables	Very high
Fruit	Very high
Sweets	Nil

48

Choline

Common name

Choline.

Alternative names

Amantine. Bilineurine. Neurine. Gossypine. Vidine.
Chicken antiperosis factor. Vitamin B_p.
Lipid mobiliser. Fat-fighter. Anti-fat agent.

Betaine (trimethylglycine) is a derivative.

History

1862: The compound was first isolated from lecithin from bile by Strecker and called choline.

1865: The compound called neurine, found in brain, was synthesized by Liebreich.

1898: Neurine and choline were shown to be identical, and the name choline was adopted. Around that time, lecithin was characterized chemically as phosphatidylcholine.

1921: The first neurotransmitter to be discovered was acetylcholine in 1921, for which Loewi and Hallett earned the Nobel Prize in 1936.

1954: Kennedy described the cytidine 5-dihphosphocholine pathway by which choline is incorporated into phosphatidylcholine.

1960: A second route, the phosphatidylethanolamine-N-methyltransferase pathway, was identified by Bremer and Greenberg.

1998: One hundred years later, choline was classified as an essential nutrient.

There are nine members of the B-group vitamins as listed in Fig. 48.1.

Fig. 48.1. The B-Group Vitamins

- Choline ----------
- Niacin (Vitamin B_3)
- Pantothenic Acid (Vitamin B_5)
- Vitamin B_6 (Pyridoxine)
- Riboflavin (Vitamin B_2)
- Thiamine (Vitamin B_1)
- Folate (Vitamin B_9)
- Biotin (Vitamin B_7)
- Vitamin B_{12} (Cobalamin)

Each of these will be considered in detail in the following chapters.

Nature

Choline is a quaternary amino cationic organic alcohol. Choline is a water-soluble vitamin-like conditionally essential nutrient usually included with the B-group vitamins. Choline is an absolutely essential nutrient for humans when excess methionine and folate are not available in the diet. Choline is widely distributed in plants and animals. It occurs in the phospholipid, lecithin, and also in the nerve transmitter acetylcholine. Free choline occurs as a trimethylammonium salt.

Biological Functions

- Choline is involved primarily with the utilization of lipids and cholesterol in the body. It prevents the accumulation of fat in the liver by promoting its transport. The relative biopotency of choline and some derivatives to inhibit deposition or to hasten removal of excessive amounts of fat from the liver is given in Table 48.1. In animals, the ability to prevent haemorrhagic kidney damage follows a similar pattern.

- Choline is used in the synthesis of the phospholipids, phosphatidylcholine and sphingomyelin which contribute to the structural integrity of cell membranes.

- About 95% of total choline in tissues is in the form of phosphatidylcholines (lecithins).

- Lecithin may help to prevent the formation of gallstones.

- The choline-containing phospholipids are precursors for diacylglycerol and ceramide which are involved in cell signaling.

- Platelet activating factor and sphingophosphocholine are other cell signaling metabolites containing choline.

- Choline, together with the amino acid methionine, is involved in the transfer of methyl groups ($-CH_3$) by a process called transmethylation.

- Choline is required for the synthesis of acetylcholine. Acetylcholine is involved in many functions including muscle control, circadian rhythm and memory. Acetylcholine is a neurotransmitter in the autonomic nervous system and at neuromuscular junctions.

- Choline is essential for maintaining the nerve cell coverings. These so-called myelin sheaths cover the long processes called axons of nerve cells and, thus, aid in the transmission of nervous impulses.

- In some animals, choline is essential for optimal brain development.

- In humans, there is little evidence to show that choline supplementation during pregnancy improves an infant's cognitive ability.

- The role of choline in possibly preventing cognitive decline in older people is uncertain.

- It is not yet known whether high plasma levels of choline during pregnancy can protect against neurotubular defects.

- Choline catalyses the remethylation of homocysteine to methionine.

- The metabolic pathways of choline, methionine, folate and vitamin B_{12} overlap and help resist infection.

- Choline is oxidised to betaine in the liver and kidney. The choline metabolite, betaine, is involved in the regulation of homocysteine concentration in the blood. Betaine contributes up to 60% of the methyl groups required for the methylation of homocysteine.

- In several studies, choline exerts a strong lipotropic effect and betaine exerts a moderate lipotropic effect. Both may help to repair alcohol-induced fatty liver damage.

- Betaine is an osmoregulator especially in the kidney.

- CDP-choline (cytidine diphosphocholine, also called citicoline) another choline derivative, stimulates the synthesis of the catecholamines, which include noradrenaline, adrenaline, and dopamine, all of which are derivatives of tyrosine.

- Supplementation with CDP-choline may help to limit neurologic damage in stroke patients and may be effective in Parkinson's disease.

- Choline may strengthen the walls of capillary vessels, and has been used therapeutically to improve blood flow to the eyes.

- CDP-choline may improve retinal function in some glaucoma patients.

Requirement

The daily intake of choline in the average Western diet is in the range 500 to 1,000 mg. The daily requirement of choline in males is 550 mg/d and in females is 425 mg/d, respectively. Therapeutic doses range from 0.5 to 6.0 grams per day. Choline is required in the diet, even though it is synthesised in the liver. Phosphatidylethanolamine is converted into phosphatidylcholine in the presence of folate and vitamin B_{12}, but it is not synthesized fast enough to provide all the human needs. Good dietary sources of choline include egg yolks, liver, meat, poultry and fish, and several fruits and vegetables, including figs, avocados, brussels sprouts and cauliflower. Further details are given in the compendium (Table 48.2). The best source of betaine is wheat, especially bran.

Toxicity

There is no toxicity associated with choline in the diet. Massive doses, if prolonged, may deplete vitamin B_6. The tolerable upper intake level for adults is 3.5 g/day. Excessive consumption of choline, greater than 7.5 grams, can have a number of effects, such as lowering blood pressure, lightheadedness, excessive sweating, salivation, a fishy body odor caused by trimethylamine, and gastrointestinal disturbances.

Deficiency

Signs of choline deficiency include increased liver enzymes and an elevated enzyme, called creatine phosphokinase (CPK), indicating muscle damage. In experimental animals, deficiency results in impaired lipid mobilization and transport, resulting in fatty livers. Without adequate phosphatidylcholine, fat and cholesterol accumulates in the liver. Fatty livers do not generally occur during a choline deficiency in the presence of adequate protein in the diet. Prolonged choline deficiency may cause ulcers. Choline deficiency in pregnant women can result in elevated levels of the amino acid homocysteine. This can be toxic to fetuses and may increases the risk of birth defects. In animals, haemorrhagic kidney necrosis and anaemia have been observed, but these effects have not been observed in humans. Vitamin B_{12} deficiency interferes with the synthesis of choline. In certain cases, deficiency has been implicated with high blood pressure and atherosclerosis. Other symptoms include fatigue, nerve damage, faulty memory and mood changes.

Table 48.1. Relative lipotropic and antihaemorrhagic biopotency of choline and some derivatives

NAME	NOMINAL VALUE (relative effect)	RELATIVE POTENCY (percent)
Choline	Strong effect	100
Betaine	Moderate effect	33
CDP-Choline	Weak effect	3

myo-Inositol also has a weak lipotropic effect.

Table 48.2. Choline compendium

FOOD GROUP	CHOLINE LEVEL
Milk and products	Low
Eggs	Low
Meat and fish	Very variable
Fats and oils	Nil
Grain and products	Medium, variable
Nuts and pulses	High
Root vegetables	Very low
Leaf vegetables	Medium, variable
Fruit	Very low, variable
Sweets	Nil

49

Niacin

Common Names

Niacin.
Nicotinamide.
Vitamin B_3.

Alternative Names

Nicotinic acid amide. Nicotinamide. Niacinamide.
Vitamin PP (Pellagra Preventative). Antipellagra vitamin.
PP Factor. Energy Vitamin. B_3, B_4 and occasionally B_7.
3-Pyridine-carboxylic acid. Pyridine-β–carboxylic acid.
Canine anti-black tongue factor.

Many of the above terms are now obsolete.

History

-----: Pellagra has been known for centuries.

1735: Pellagra was first described as a disease by Casal.

circa 1800: Marzari correlated pellagra with some form of inadequacy in a maize diet.

1867: Huber oxidised nicotine and isolated nicotinic acid.

circa 1913: Nicotinic acid isolated by Funk, and also by Suzuki, from rice polishings and yeast.

1915: Goldberger demonstrated that pellagra was a nutritional deficiency and not, as had previously been thought; a disease caused by infection.

1917: Chittenden and Underhill showed that canine black tongue is similar to human pellagra.

circa 1935: Warburg and Christian find that nicotinamide is a part of the old Coenzyme II, now called NADP. About the same time Kuhn and Vetter isolate nicotinamide from heart muscle.

circa 1936: Von Euler, *et al.*, discover another coenzyme contains nicotinamide. This coenzyme, previously called Coenzyme I, is now called NAD. Von Euler also determines the structure of NAD, in 1936.

1937: Elvehjem, *et al.*, find that nicotinamide was the active principle in liver which cured black tongue in dogs. Late in the same year it was reported by Fouts, *et al.*, that nicotinamide cures pellagra in humans.

1945: Krehl, *et al.*, found that tryptophan can be substituted for the vitamin niacin.

1947: Handily and Bond establish the conversion of tryptophan to nicotinic acid in animals.

1949: It was shown the tryptophan could also be converted into nicotinic acid in humans.

-----: Niacin is now a generic term for nicotinic acid and nicotinamide. The measure, Niacin Equivalents, includes the contribution of tryptophan to the total vitamin activity.

Nature

Niacin is synthesised by higher plants and most bacteria, but the extent to which niacin is available from the gut bacteria is unknown. Niacin may also be synthesised from the essential amino acid tryptophan in many animals including humans. However, the synthesis from tryptophan is usually insufficient to provide the full daily requirement and hence niacin is considered to be a conditionally essential vitamin in humans.

There are two natural interconvertible forms of niacin namely, nicotinic acid and nicotinamide. Chemically, nicotinic acid is a pyridine ring carboxylated at position 3. The amide contains the – $CONH_2$ group instead of the –COOH group in the same position. The term niacin is now used as a generic descriptor for both nicotinic acid and nicotinamide rather than as a synonym for just nicotinic acid. The term Niacin Equivalent (NE), however, is officially used as a quantitative measure for all substances with nicotinic acid activity, and therefore includes the contribution made by tryptophan. On average 1 mg niacin can be derived from 60 mg tryptophan in the body. Put another way, 100 mg tryptophan may contribute 1.7 mg niacin. Niacin is a very stable vitamin. The potencies of niacin and tryptophan are summarised in Table 49.1.

There are two coenzyme forms of niacin, namely nicotinamide adenine dinucleotide, or NAD for short (previously termed Coenzyme I), and nicotinamide adenine dinucleotide phosphate, or NADP for short (previously termed Coenzyme II). The only difference between these two coenzymes is one extra phosphate group in NADP. NAD is a complex molecule consisting of nicotinamide linked to ribose which in turn is linked to two phosphate links attached to adenosine (which consists of adenine and ribose). In NADP, an extra phosphate is attached to the adenosine ribose.

Biological Functions

- The coenzyme, NAD, is chiefly involved with tissue oxidation (catabolism) of substances to release energy, whereas the coenzyme, NADP, is chiefly involved with synthetic (anabolic) reactions, particularly those involving lipid and steroid metabolism.

- Both coenzymes undergo reversible oxidation and reduction – hence, their vital role in the hydrogen and electron transport systems which are essential for cell respiration.

- The NAD form serves as an electron and hydrogen carrier in the mitochondria, where it helps to trap the high energy of free electrons and couple it to the formation of adenosine triphosphate, ATP, in a process called oxidative phosphorylation.

- Both NAD and NADP are involved in electron transport in the liver microsomes which are responsible for the hydroxylation of various drugs including steroids in the body.

- Together, therefore, the two coenzyme forms of niacin are extensively involved in all aspects of metabolism including, glycolysis, pyruvate metabolism, pentose metabolism, lipid including steroid metabolism, oxidative deamination, and the synthesis of high energy phosphates including ATP.

- The amino acid, tryptophan, may be converted to nicotinic acid in the body.

- Nicotinic acid and nicotinamide are interconvertible in the body by a series of reactions involving NAD itself as an intermediate.

- Large doses of nicotinic acid result in a lowered blood cholesterol by an unknown mechanism and may inhibit the formation of blood clots. Nicotinamide does not seem to have this therapeutic property to the same extent.

- Large doses of nicotinamide result in increased concentrations of NAD in the liver.

- Nicotinamide tends to deflect methyl groups ($-CH_3$) away from choline synthesis. Such substances have been termed antilipotropic because they tend to reduce lipid mobilisation in the body, and hence the overall lipid levels in the blood.

- A phosphorylated form of NAD (not the same as NADP) is formed in heart muscle during hydrogen transport from succinic acid. In the presence of magnesium this intermediate helps to phosphorylate ADP to ATP with the liberation of NAD.

- Through its various metabolic roles, niacin helps to maintain healthy tissues, including the skin, the tongue, the brain and other nervous tissue, and the digestive system.

- Niacin may participate in certain non-oxidative reactions in the body.

- Niacin in high does may alleviate the symptoms of

schizophrenia in certain patients. High dosage, or megavitamin therapy, with niacin has also produced some good results in treating alcoholics, heart patients, and mentally disturbed children.

Requirement

The requirement for niacin is believed by many nutritionists to be related to energy expenditure. This is because of its extensive involvement in metabolic processes. The amount of niacin required per 1,000 kcal has been estimated to be about 6.6 (and occasionally as high as 7.2 mg) niacin equivalents (NE). In modern energy units, this value translates to give about 1.6 mg NE per 1,000 kilojoules.

In the typical Western diet, some 36 percent of the niacin requirement comes from meat and fish, another 20 percent comes from grain products, and 14 percent each are provided by milk products and vegetables, respectively. A compendium is also included here for reference (Table 49.2). Niacin in grain is often bound in a form called niacytin. In this form, it is largely unavailable in the diet, and this can lead to unexpected deficiencies. Treatment with alkali before cooking can render this form available, as is the practice in certain parts of Mexico. Unless this is done, corn for example is inadequate because it is also very low in tryptophan. It is believed that an unbalanced amino acid intake may also lead to niacin deficiencies. For example, in India a grain called sorghum is a major crop. This cereal has a high leucine to isoleucine ratio, and leads to niacin deficiencies if not supplemented in the diet.

In theory, because of the possible conversion of tryptophan to niacin in the body, it is possible to provide the full dietary requirement for niacin by substituting sufficient tryptophan. It requires one gram of tryptophan to supply the daily requirement of niacin for a typical adult. But this amount is subject to individual variation because the extent of conversion is not a fixed value. But the overall ratio of 60 mg tryptophan yielding 1 mg niacin is an average value which has now been accepted by definition. On average, about 1.4 grams of tryptophan are provided by 100 grams of animal protein and around

1.0 gram of tryptophan is provided by 100 grams of vegetable protein. As a matter of interest, the conversion of tryptophan to nicotinic acid requires vitamin B_6 as a cofactor. Therefore, if vitamin B_6 is deficient, the niacin equivalency of tryptophan may be incomplete or absent.

In general, an absolute minimum adult dose of 10 mg niacin per day is required to prevent the onset of pellagra. However, this amount is not considered sufficient for optimum health or to fully maintain adequate stores of niacin in the body. It has been found that daily intakes between 11 and 13 NE in adults are required to maintain the body stores. Niacin may be stored for short periods in the liver, but excess is rapidly lost in the urine. The human requirement for niacin is increased during pregnancy and lactation. The recommended daily intake of niacin in males is 16 mg/d and in females is 14 mg/d, respectively. The average intake of pre-formed niacin in the typical Western diet is around 8 to 17 mg niacin equivalents per day. This is supplemented by potential niacin in the form of 600 to 1,200 mg tryptophan, supplying an additional 10 to 20 mg niacin equivalents.

Toxicity

Niacin is a relatively non-toxic substance because it is rapidly eliminated in the urine when present in excess. Intakes up to 50 mg in children or 100 mg in adults generally produce no side effects. However, even relatively small doses (as little as 100 µg) of nicotinic acid may produce sudden vasodilation and flushing of the skin on the face, upper body, and even more extensively, which may last for 10 to 15 minutes. Sometimes, this is accompanied by a feeling of surface heat and occasionally by a throbbing headache. But the effect is generally considered therapeutic in promoting circulation and in temporarily lowering blood pressure. Regular use of supplementary nicotinic acid also lowers blood cholesterol which is an important side effect. The pure nicotinamide form does not have these effects to the same extent, if at all. One gram or more of nicotinic acid may, apart from the above-mentioned symptoms, produce stomach cramps, nausea and diarrhoea. These effects of nicotinic acid may be augmented in patients on certain antibiotics. On the other hand, regular intakes of high doses of the acid form will diminish the intensity of the flushing effect. Indeed, sequential dosing with 100 mg tablets may not elicit further symptoms. A single dose of 2 to 3 grams of the nicotinamide form may produce toxic effects in the liver. Excessive intake of niacin may cause an imbalance in the other members of the B-group vitamins. Some individuals have been known to take up to 4 grams of nicotinic acid per day over long periods without toxic effects. But on 6 grams per day, some individuals may develop mild symptoms of gout, itching, boils and skin rashes. The nicotinic acid form may sometimes irritate stomach ulcers in certain patients.

It is reported that one individual once tried to commit suicide with nicotinic acid. He swallowed 90 grams of the vitamin but only succeeded in making himself very nauseous which was accompanied by a bout of vomiting and a bad dose of diarrhoea.

Deficiency

Excessive consumption of carbohydrates may deplete the body stores of niacin. Certain antibiotics can have the same effect. In the early stages of deficiency, there occurs a generalised weakness, loss of appetite, some gastric disturbances and skin lesions (canker sores). Irritability, nausea, and vomiting, frequently occur, and headaches and ulcerous sores may also develop. In the full-blown condition called pellagra, a deep depression may develop leading to dementia. This dementia together with the dermatitis and diarrhoea completes the characteristic Three D's typical of pellagra. Nervous disorders and tremors may occur and the mouth and gums become inflamed. The tongue may be swollen, dark red and sore. Hence the expression blacktongue, used to describe the condition in niacin deficient dogs. Gradually the mucous membranes throughout the body including the gastrointestinal tract will become inflamed and haemorrhagic.

Some of the abovementioned symptoms may reflect a contemporary deficiency of other B-group vitamins and proteins in the diet. There may be a skin sensitivity to sunlight, and a severe dehydration is common. Haemolytic anaemia may develop and ultimately death will result unless the condition is treated. Strange as it may seem, no serious impairment of oxidative reactions catalysed by NAD or NADP occur, even in severely deficient states. Hence, the symptoms of pellagra are not fully explainable in terms of the expected metabolic lesions. Pellagra rapidly responds to treatment with niacin. Dramatic improvements can usually be observed after just one day. The drug isonicotinic acid hydrazide (or isoniazid) is a potent vitamin B_6 antagonist. Patients treated with this drug (used for tuberculosis) frequently develop symptoms of niacin deficiency. This is because vitamin B_6 is essential for the conversion of tryptophan to nicotinic acid in the body. This is an important additional source of the vitamin and in its absence, sufficient niacin may not be available from the diet. A rare genetic defect of tryptophan transport called Hartnup disease (pellagra-like dermatosis) causes the same effects but may be corrected by administering large doses of niacin. Niacin deficiency generally develops after 50 to 60 days in persons maintained on an unsupplemented corn diet. In experimental niacin-tryptophan deficiency studies, the urinary excretion of niacin decreases rapidly in the first 30 days and generally reaches a minimal value after about 60 days. Thereafter clinical symptoms of deficiency become evident.

Table 49.1. Relative biopotency of different forms of niacin and tryptophan

NAME	NOMINAL VALUE (percent)
Nicotinic acid	100
Nicotinamide	100
NAD	19
NADP	17
Tryptophan	1.7
Trigonelline	0

Trigonelline is a methylated form of nicotinic acid found in some seeds. Because of their larger size, the coenzymes of niacin have relatively lower potencies. Theoretical values for NAD and NADP are given above.

Table 49.2. Niacin compendium

FOOD GROUP	NIACIN LEVEL
Milk and products	Very low
Eggs	Very low
Meat and fish	Very variable
Fats and oils	Nil
Grain and products	Very high
Nuts and pulses	Very high, variable
Root vegetables	Medium
Leaf vegetables	Medium
Fruit	Low
Sweets	Very low, variable

50
Pantothenic Acid

Common name

Pantothenic Acid.
Vitamin B$_5$.

Alternative names

D-Pantothenic acid. Pantothenate. Pantoyl moiety.
Pantoyl-β–alanine.
Yeast growth factor. Growth promoter (for bacteria).
Rat liver filtrate factor.
Chick antidermatitis factor. Antidermatitis vitamin.
Anti-grey hair factor. Anti-stress vitamin.
Vitamin B$_3$ and occasionally B$_x$.

Many of the above terms are obsolete.

History

1901: Wilders gives the name Bios to a cell-free yeast extract that promotes growth in yeast. Subsequently, Bios is shown to contain several substances as follows: in 1920, Bios I (now called inositol); in 1933, Bios IIA (now called pantothenic acid); and in 1936, Bios IIB (now called biotin.)

1933: Williams isolates and crystallises Bios IIA from yeast and names it pantothenic acid, because it is an acidic substance and widely distributed.

circa 1938: Snell, *et al.,* establishes pantothenic acid as a growth promoter for lactic acid bacteria. In the same year, Williams isolates a factor from a liver filtrate.

1939: Jukes shows that the liver factor which prevents dermatitis in chickens is the same as the yeast factor, namely pantothenic acid. Wolley shows that pantothenic acid contains β–alanine.

1940: Harris, *et al.*, determine the structure, synthesise, and crystallise pantothenic acid.

circa 1947: Lipmann, *et al.*, discover that CoA (first identified as a heat stable coenzyme in 1945) contains pantothenic acid.

1951: Lynen, fully characterises the structure of CoA.

1965: Wakil, *et al.* and Majerus, *et al.*, discover 4-phospho-pantheteine to be a key component of the acyl carrier protein complex.

Nature

Pantothenic acid can be synthesised in higher plants and in many microorganisms, however the availability of pantothenic acid from the gut bacteria is unknown. There is only one natural form of pantothenic acid, although a number of synthetic forms have been studied in recent years. Pantothenic acid is simple molecule which is made up of pantoic acid linked to beta-alanine. Neither pantoic acid nor β–alanine have any vitamin activity in humans. The biopotencies of different forms of pantothenic acid are given in Table 50.1.

Pantothenic acid is also a component of the vital coenzyme called Coenzyme A, or CoA for short. This coenzyme consists of pantothenic acid linked to thioethanolamine (previously termed mercaptoethylamine) at its β–alanine end, and at its pantoic end to a double phosphate link which connects to a phosphorylated adenosine unit (much in the same way as NADP, considered in the previous Chapter). The thiol side of the molecule ends in a sulfhydryl group (– SH).

Biological Functions

- Pantothenic acid is a component of acyl carrier protein (ACP), which forms a key part of a multienzyme complex (involving seven separate functions) associated with fatty acid synthesis.

The form in which the vitamin occurs there is 4-phosphopantheteine. This may be considered the simplest coenzyme form of the vitamin and consists chemically of pantothenic acid linked at its β–alanine end to a single phosphate group. The entire complex is called fatty acid synthase and occurs in the cytoplasm of all cells. Its main function is to catalyze the synthesis of fatty acids, such as palmitate, from acetyl-CoA and malonyl-CoA.

- At the thiol end of the molecule, the sulfhydryl group (–SH) may react with acyl groups to form high energy metabolic intermediates such as active acetate. Acyl groups (RCO–) are all functional derivatives of fatty acids. Such intermediates are essential in acetylation reactions, the metabolism of fatty acids, ketone bodies and steroids and, together with thiamine pyrophosphate, in oxidative decarboxylation of carbohydrates and amino acids. They derive their energy from ATP or equivalent energy stores.

- CoA is involved extensively in all aspects of metabolism and it cooperates with other vitamins in many reactions. Indeed, over 70 reactions are now known which require CoA. Coenzyme A, therefore serves a fundamental role in metabolism by activating and transporting a large number of organic groups such as acetate, propionate, crotonate, malonate, succinate, citrate, benzoate, choline, and many others.

- Pantothenic acid assists in the formation of haem, the essential component of haemoglobin, the oxygen carrying protein in the red blood cell.

- Pantothenic acid is involved in the production of acetylcholine which is one of the major nerve and muscle transmitter substances.

- Pantothenic acid protects against infections by promoting the formation of antibodies in the blood.

- Pantothenic acid reduces some toxic effects associated with exposure to radiation.

- Pantothenic acid may help to detoxify certain antibiotics such as sulphanilamide.

- Pantothenic acid may protect against some of the side effects of alcohol abuse.

- Pantothenic acid may help the body to cope with tiredness and stress and it is claimed that it helps maintain the youthful appearance of skin and hair.

- Pantothenic acid administered in high doses to rats increases their life-span.

Requirement

Pantothenic acid is widely distributed particularly in animal tissues such as liver and kidney where it derives from plant sources. Other good sources include milk, eggs, yeast and whole grain products. A compendium is included which indicates further dietary sources of pantothenic acid (Table 50.2). The average intake of pantothenic acid per day varies widely but is usually in the range 5 to 20 mg. About half of this is in the free form and the other half is conjugated. An intake of 5 mg in most adults is sufficient to maintain pantothenic acid balance in the body. However, higher values have been suggested for pregnant and lactating women.

Toxicity

Pantothenic acid has no known toxic effects. The therapeutic use of supplements up to 1,000 mg per day in some patients over a six-month period had no obvious side effects. However, excessive intake may cause an imbalance of other B-group vitamins and, in some cases, mild intestinal distress and diarrhea. Some authors claim that under stressful conditions the optimum intake may even be as high as 30 - 50 mg per day in some individuals. Occasionally, up to ten times these amounts have been suggested. In fact, treatment with 2,000 mg per for two months in a number of arthritic patients resulted in some improvement in their symptoms.

Deficiency

A deficiency of pantothenic acid hardly ever occurs. A deficiency may contribute to the burning feet syndrome, where the feet become very sore or painful accompanied by a sensation of burning. Other signs of deficiency are more general and include loss of appetite, muscular cramps, neuritis, and a tendency towards upper respiratory infections. Mental depression and insomnia may occur in severe deficiency states, leading possibly to frank psychosis. Heavy drinkers tend to be deficient in pantothenic acid as well as a range of other vitamins. Arthritic patients tend to have low blood levels of pantothenic acid. Allergic reactions are often more intense in pantothenic acid deficient patients, and they may have a decreased capacity for antibody formation. A sensitivity to the hormone insulin may develop. Many of the symptoms of pantothenic acid deficiency are consequent upon a general slowing down of metabolism. In certain animals, deficiency symptoms include degeneration of the neuromuscular structures, adrenaline insufficiency, and ultimately death. In persons maintained without pantothenic acid only vague feelings of deficiency were noticed. After about 70 days a sense of fatigue was reported but the burning feet syndrome did not occur at that stage.

Table 50.1. Relative biopotency of pantothenic acid
and related compounds

NAME	NOMINAL VALUE (percent)
Pantothenic Acid	100
Dexpanthenol	107
Pantothenyl alcohol	85
4-phosphopantheteine	70
CoA	70
Pantoic Acid	0
β–Alanine	0

Because of their relatively larger size the coenzymes of pantothenic acid have relatively lower potencies. The values for 4-phosphopantheteine and CoA are theoretical. Pantothenyl alcohol is a synthetic form and has relative activity in some tests.

Table 50.2. Pantothenic acid compendium

FOOD GROUP	PANTOTHENIC ACID LEVEL
Milk and products	Medium, variable
Eggs	High
Meat and fish	Very variable
Fats and oils	Very low
Grain and products	High, variable
Nuts and pulses	High, variable
Root vegetables	Medium
Leaf vegetables	High
Fruit	Very low
Sweets	Nil

51

Vitamin B6

Common names

Vitamin B6
Pyridoxine.

Alternative names

B6 group. Pyridoxal. Pyridoxamine. Aldermin or Aldermine. Pyridoxol (hydrochloride). Antidermatitis factor. Antiacrodynia factor. Anti-depression vitamin. Yeast eluate factor. Factor Y. Factor I. H.

Many of the above terms are obsolete or trivial.

History

1926: Goldberger and Lillie produced a form of dermatitis in rats on a diet deficient in a certain factor.

1934: The existence of a new B Vitamin distinct from niacin or riboflavin was recognised and defined as a cure for rat dermatitis by Paul György, who proposed the name Vitamin B6 This extract was obtained from yeast.

1936: The structure of Vitamin B6 was partially characterised by Birch and György.

1938: Lepkovsky isolated a similar factor from rice bran. Keresztesy and Stevens crystallised pure Vitamin B6 from rice polishings. In the same year Kohn, *et al.*, synthesised one form of Vitamin B6 and called it pyridoxine.

1939: Stiller, *et al.*, established the structure of pyridoxine.

1944: Pyridoxal and Pyridoxamine were discovered to be alternative forms of Vitamin B_6, by Snell.

1945 *et seq.*: Snell proposed that some form might be part of a coenzyme for transamination reactions. Subsequently, the active forms of Vitamin B_6 were discovered to be phosphorylated derivatives of pyridoxine. Pyridoxal phosphate is the principle form. Pyridoxamine phosphate also occurs.

1953: Snyderman, *et al.*, established full recognition of the human requirement for Vitamin B_6

-----: Vitamin B_6 is now a generic term for all 3–hydroxy–2–methyl-pyridine derivatives that exhibit qualitatively the biological activity of pyridoxine.

Nature

Vitamin B_6 is synthesised in higher plants and many microorganisms, and some of the vitamin requirement as supplied by the gut bacteria. The term vitamin B_6 is now used as a generic descriptor for all 2-methylpyridine derivatives with pyridoxine activity. The vitamin also occurs in animals although it is not synthesised by them. There are three equally active natural forms of vitamin B_6 namely, pyridoxine, pyridoxal and pyridoxamine. Pyridoxine is the chief plant form and is usually taken as the most representative compound of the vitamin B_6 group, although the main forms occurring in animal tissues are pyridoxal and pyridoxamine. Pyridoxic acid is a breakdown product and is inactive.

Like niacin, vitamin B_6 chemically consists of derivatives of the pyridine ring structure. All natural forms have a methyl (–CH_3) group on position 2, a hydroxyl (–OH) group on position 3, and a hydroxymethyl (–CH_2OH) group on position 5. They differ according to the group attached to position 4. In the case of pyridoxine this group is another hydromethyl group. For pyridoxal the group is an aldehyde (–CHO). For pyridoxamine the group is an amide (–CH_2NH_2). And for pyridoxic acid the group is a carboxyl (–COOH). Table 51.1 summarises the biopotencies of a number of vitamin B_6 compounds. Vitamin B_6 is a very stable vitamin.

Biological Functions

- There are three interconvertible phosphorylated coenzyme forms of vitamin B_6, namely pyridoxine phosphate, pyridoxal phosphate and pyridoxamine phosphate. Like biotin, these vitamin B_6 coenzymes are linked through epsilon-amino groups of lysine to various enzymes. During reactions, the ε–link is replaced by α–amino groups of various amino acids which undergo a variety of important reactions. Pyridoxal phosphate requires the activity of an enzyme called pyridoxal kinase to form it directly in the cell. However, pyridoxine phosphate may be converted to pyridoxal phosphate by the action of a flavoprotein. Subsequently, pyridoxal phosphate and pyridoxamine phosphate are interconvertible.

- Vitamin B_6 dependent enzymes are essential in decarboxylation reactions and in nitrogen and sulphur metabolism. In their absence, substrates buildup such as homocysteine (which is normally converted to cysteine) and may appear in the urine. During metabolism of amino acids to keto acids and *vice versa*, the coenzyme pyridoxal phosphate is converted to pyridoxamine phosphate and then back again. As a result, one amino acid and one keto acid are converted into a different amino acid and a different keto acid, respectively.

- The various reactions involving vitamin B_6 as a coenzyme include decarboxylations (which involve the removal of carboxyl groups, –COOH); deaminations (where amino groups, –NH_2, are removed from amino acids); transaminations (where such groups are transferred to form different amino acids); desulphurations (here sulfhydryl groups, –SH, are removed); transsulphurations (where such groups are transferred to form a different sulfur containing amino acid) and racemisations (which involve molecular rearrangements).

- Vitamin B_6 promotes the transport of amino acids into cells and consequently their metabolic utilization as considered above.

- Through its metabolic roles, vitamin B_6 helps maintain the health of muscle tissue including the heart, the nervous system, and the skin.

- Vitamin B_6 may be beneficial in the treatment of early morning sickness during pregnancy in some women. The dose should not exceed 25 mg per day in these circumstances because of the risk to the foetus.

- Vitamin B_6 may also be beneficial in the treatment of premenstrual tension. Here it may help to maintain the proper distribution of sodium and potassium and consequently the fluid balance in the body. It is believed that the temporary increase in the hormone estrogen around this time may interfere with normal absorption or utilization of vitamin B_6. Estrogen is also a component in the contraceptive pill and prolonged use of such pills may lower the vitamin B_6 levels in the blood. Supplements of 50 to 100 mg per day have been used to offset this effect.

- Vitamin B_6 is involved in the formation of haemoglobin. It probably acts through its roles in the metabolism of amino acids and in the absorption of vitamin B_{12}.

- Vitamin B_6 is essential for the metabolism of tryptophan which gives rise to another vitamin namely niacin in the body.

- Vitamin B_6 is essential for the formation of serotonin in the pineal gland in the brain. It may therefore be of benefit in the treatment of insomnia in certain individuals. Serotonin also helps to counteract the effects of mental depression.

- Vitamin B_6 can form uncharged chelates (complexes) with certain mineral ions. These are stable in both aqueous and lipid media and therefore aid in the active transport of such minerals across cell membranes.

- Vitamin B_6 is involved in the synthesis of adrenaline. Consequently, it helps in the utilization of glycogen and its release from the liver stores when required.

- Vitamin B_6 promotes the utilization of linoleic acid in the body, and the formation of long-chain polyunsaturated fatty acids.

- Vitamin B_6 promotes the absorption of vitamin B_{12}, and has a role to play in maintaining an adequate production of hydrochloric acid (HCl) in the stomach.

- Vitamin B_6 may protect against some of the effects of alcohol abuse.

- Vitamin B_6 is involved in the production of a number of important but lesser known intermediates in the cell including taurocholic acid, sphingomyelin and δ–aminolevulinic acid.

- Vitamin B_6 also helps in the formation of antibodies.

- Treatment with supplements of vitamin B_6 may be beneficial in certain cases of epilepsy and schizophrenia.

- It has been claimed that vitamin B_6 may aid memory and dream recall.

Requirement

Vegetables, meat and grain products are excellent sources of vitamin B_6. Further details are included in the compendium (Table 51.2). The requirement for vitamin B_6 is related to the intake of protein because the vitamin is essential to all aspects of amino acid metabolism in the body. Individuals on high protein diets therefore require additional vitamin B_6. The average daily intake of vitamin B_6 in typical Western diets is around 2 mg.

The metabolites of tryptophan called xanthurenic acid, kynurenine and hydroxykynurenine are excreted in the urine following a tryptophan loading test. In one study, it was found that xanthurenic acid could be normalised by administering 1.25 mg vitamin B_6 to subjects ingesting 30 grams of protein per day, or 1.50 mg vitamin B_6 to subjects ingesting 100 grams per day. In other studies, somewhat lower values were found. As a rough guide, it seems that for most adults 1.5 mg of vitamin B_6 per day is adequate with low protein intakes, and 2.0 mg per day is adequate with high protein intakes. The recommended adult daily intake of vitamin B_6 in males is 1.7 mg/d and in females is 1.5 mg/d, respectively. The requirement for vitamin B_6 increases slightly with age. There is an increased requirement for vitamin B_6 during pregnancy and lactation and also for women who take the contraceptive pill.

Toxicity

Vitamin B_6 is relatively non-toxic because excess is rapidly excreted in the urine. However, high doses may lead to toxic symptoms including restlessness at night and vivid dream recall on waking. It is not recommended to take supplements of vitamin B_6 on a regular basis. One group who took 200 mg of pyridoxine for one month became dependent on the high dose. Also, there is a risk of imbalance in other members of the B-group vitamins. Prolonged intake of high doses of vitamin B_6 may lead to peripheral neuropathy, where the most common symptoms include pain, tingling sensations in the extremities, particularly the fingers, pins and needles, and numbness. The gait may become unsteady and the lips and tongue may become numb. Toxic effects are usually manifested on intakes of 2 grams or more per day. However, it is not recommended to exceed 200 mg per day because of the risk of sensory or peripheral neuropathy. In some cases, single doses of 200-300 mg have been found to elicit some toxic symptoms. Therefore, vitamin B_6 is not quite as safe in high doses as it was once assumed to be. High doses of vitamin B_6 may counteract some actions of L-dopa. In normal people, L-dopa is an adequate precursor of noradrenaline, the sympathetic nerve transmitter. However, supplements of L-dopa may be required by certain patients with Parkinson's disease, to control their symptoms.

Deficiency

Because of the link between vitamin B_6 and the synthesis of niacin in the body, deficiency of vitamin B_6 is generally accompanied by symptoms of niacin deficiency at the same time. In some cases of kidney disease, the enzyme pyridoxal kinase is inhibited and, even though vitamin B_6 intake may be normal, the active coenzyme may not be adequately formed. Strict vegetarians may be at risk of vitamin B6 deficiency. The anti-tuberculosis drug isonicotinic acid hydride (isoniazid) is a vitamin B_6 antagonist. Treatment with this drug may produce symptoms of vitamin B_6 deficiency in persons on an otherwise normal diet.

A significant deficiency of vitamin B_6 is rare. The symptoms of deficiency can be very general including loss of weight, irritability, stomach pains and vomiting. Irregular brain waves and in extreme cases convulsions may develop. During vitamin B_6 deficiency, there is a buildup of the protein components of various pyridoxal phosphate-dependent enzymes in the liver. But these remain inactive due to lack of the required coenzyme. In rats, epilepsy my result because of nerve damage. Also in the rat, growth ceases, dermatitis develops and oedema of the tail, ears and paws may develop. In monkeys, atherosclerosis may develop.

Some individuals are known to have a dependency on vitamin B_6. In such cases, normal levels of the vitamin may be insufficient and high-dose supplementation may be necessary to prevent symptoms which may include seizures, anaemia, xanthurenic acidurea, cystathioninurea or homocystinurea. Many normal infants may develop convulsions on a vitamin deficient diet. On the other hand, some infants with a pyridoxine-dependency have a dramatically increased requirement (2 – 10 mg per day) for vitamin B_6 and may develop convulsions (pyridoxine-dependent seizures, PDS) even on a normal diet. This condition may occur in some adults also. In infants, the convulsions are relieved by administering either vitamin B_6 or γ–aminobutyric acid (GABA). It is believed that an unusual genetic variation in the enzyme glutamate decarboxylase which requires a very high concentration of pyridoxal phosphate for activity is responsible for this condition. Similarly, in rare cases, there may be defects in the enzyme called cystathioninase (or cystathionine synthase) which may lead to a buildup of cystathionine or homocystine unless high doses of vitamin B_6 are taken.

A relative deficiency of vitamin B_6 may be induced by a high intake of proteins in the diet. Vitamin B_6 deficiency has been implicated in certain types of anaemia. In most cases, this may be an indirect consequence of impaired vitamin B_{12} absorption in humans rather than a direct effect of lack of vitamin B_6. Although a type of anaemia found in certain women on the contraceptive pill only responds to treatment with vitamin B_6. This anaemia associated with vitamin B_6 deficiency is characterised by smaller than normal red blood cells which are deficient in haemoglobin (microcytic hypochromic anaemia). It has been found that women on the contraceptive pill have lower than normal levels of vitamin B_6 in their blood plasma. Similarly, they have lower than normal activity of transaminase enzymes in both red and white blood cells. And there may be an increased excretion of tryptophan metabolites in their urine. It seems that some supplementation is necessary to correct these symptoms as not sufficient vitamin B_6 may be available in the diet.

The tryptophan metabolite, xanthurenic acid, is able to combine with insulin and inactivate it. Therefore, a mild form of diabetes may occur which has been noted in certain women on the contraceptive pill and even occasionally during pregnancy. Vitamin B_6 deficiency may result in an increased oxalic acid production. Oxalic acid is very insoluble and is one factor which contributes to the formation of kidney stones. It is believed that some forms of allergy such as hay fever, asthma and skin rashes may be due either to a deficiency of vitamin B_6 or to a greater than normal dependency on the vitamin.

Mild cases of vitamin B_6 deficiency involve metabolic lesions associated with insufficient activities of the coenzyme pyridoxal-5'-phosphate, PLP. These include impaired tryptophan-niacin conversion, resulting in urinary excretion of xanthurenic acid after an oral tryptophan load and impaired transsulfuration of methionine to cysteine. PLP-dependent transaminases and glycogen phosphorylase have a role in gluconeogenesis, so deprivation of vitamin B_6 results in impaired glucose tolerance. Symptoms of vitamin B_6 deficiency include seborrhoeic dermatitis (a form of eczema that mainly affecting the scalp and face), atrophic glossitis (a painful reddened surface of the tongue with possible oral ulceration), cheilosis (also called angular cheilitis, inflamed corners of the mouth), conjunctivitis (pinkeye, an inflammation of the conjunctiva), intertrigo (inflammation in the folds of skin), and neurologic symptoms of somnolence (drowsiness), confusion, and neuropathy (due to impaired sphingosine synthesis) and sideroblastic anemia (due to impaired haem synthesis).

In the complete absence of vitamin B6 in the diet, pyridoxine in the urine is decreased and xanthurenic acid in the urine is increased after just 7 days. After 20 days, brain wave abnormalities may be detected and thereafter epilepsy may occur.

Table 51.1. Relative biopotency of different forms of vitamin B_6

NAME	NOMINAL VALUE (percent)
Pyridoxine	100
Pyridoxal	100
Pyridoxamine	100
Pyridoxine hydrochloride	82
Pyridoxine-5'-phosphate	68
Pyridoxal-5'-phosphate	68
Pyridoxamine-5'-phosphate	68
4-Pyridoxic acid	0

Pyridoxal phosphate is considered the active form of the vitamin, while all the other forms are considered inactive as such. However, these forms are interconvertible in the body, hence they are all ultimately potent. Because of their larger size, the coenzymes have relatively lower potencies (on a weight basis) with theoretical values of approximately 65 percent on the above scale.

Table 51.2. Vitamin B_6 compendium

FOOD GROUP	VITAMIN B_6 LEVEL
Milk and products	Low, variable
Eggs	Medium
Meat and fish	Very high, variable
Fats and oils	Nil
Grain and products	Low, variable
Nuts / Pulses	Very high, variable / Low
Root vegetables	Medium
Leaf vegetables	Medium, variable
Fruit	Low, variable
Sweets	Nil

52
Riboflavin

Common name

Riboflavin.
Vitamin B$_2$.

Alternative Names

Riboflavine. Lactoflavine. Lactoflavin.
Vitamin G. Cytoflav. Ovoflavin. Hepatoflavin. Uroflavin.
Lyochrome.
Old Yellow Enzyme factor.
Anti-cheilosis vitamin.
Antidermatitis vitamin.
Energy Vitamin.

Many of the above terms are obsolete.

History

-----: For years, a rare form of facial dermatitis characterised by cracked lips and sometimes cataracts of the eyes went unrecognised as a deficiency disease of riboflavin.

1879: Blyth isolated a fluorescent yellow substance from whey.

1926: Around this time, it was believed that the vitamin B group consisted of a B$_1$ which cured beriberi and a 'B$_2$' which cured pellagra. Later, it was realised that 'B$_2$' represented several components of which niacin was the anti-pellagra vitamin.

circa 1927: Paul György and Wagner-Jauregg commenced isolating pure 'B$_2$' in order to test it on egg-white injured rats.
(At that time, dermatitis was a common feature of pellagra and its cause (egg-white injury) was subsequently shown to be due to the

lack of another vitamin, biotin.)

1932: Paul György and Wagner-Jauregg obtained a crystalline extract of 'B$_2$' from eggs which promoted growth in rats. About the same time, Warburg and Christian discovered that Old Yellow Enzyme contained a flavin as a coenzyme.

1933: Together with Kuhn, Paul György *et al.*, determine the structure of the vitamin now called riboflavin. They isolate it from other sources including whey. It was quickly found that several factors were one and the same substance. These included Cytoflav (Banga and Szent-Györgyi), Lyochrome (Ellinger and Koschara), Lactoflavin (Ellinger), and Ovoflavin (Wagner-Jauregg, *et al.*).

1934: Riboflavin was synthesised independently by Karrer, and by Kuhn, *et al.*

1938: By this time, Theorell had shown that Old Yellow Enzyme contained riboflavin-5'-phosphate, a coenzyme now called Flavin Mononucleotide (FMN). In 1938, Warburg and Christian discovered another coenzyme distinct from FMN, in an enzyme which oxidises amino acids.

1954: Todd established that this second coenzyme was Flavin Adenine Dinucleotide (FAD), and confirmed the structure by synthesising it.

Nature

Riboflavin is synthesised by higher plants and most microorganisms, but the extent of its availability from the gut bacteria is largely unknown. There is only one natural form of riboflavin although a number of synthetic derivatives have been studied in recent years. Chemically, riboflavin consists of an isoalloxazine nucleus which consists of three fused rings with the central ring linked to a D-ribitol moiety which is a derivative of the five-carbon sugar, ribose. In the presence of ultraviolet light, riboflavin is irreversibly broken down to lumiflavin (in alkaline conditions) or to lumichrome (in acidic conditions). Otherwise, riboflavin is a relatively stable compound. Neither lumiflavin or lumichrome have any vitamin activity. The biopotencies of different forms of riboflavin are given in Table 52.1.

There are two coenzyme forms of riboflavin namely, flavin mononucleotide, FMN (previously termed riboflavin phosphate), and flavin adenine dinucleotide, FAD. In FMN, riboflavin is linked to the nucleotide ribitol phosphate. In FAD, an additional component called adenosine monophosphate, AMP, is linked to the structure. The AMP moiety provides a second nucleotide, hence the term dinucleotide for this form. This second nucleotide contains an adenine unit.

Biological Functions

- There are no known functions of riboflavin in the human body other the those involving its coenzyme forms.

- In many respects, the structure of FAD resembles the structure of NAD which was considered in the chapter on niacin (Chapter 49). Also, the function of FAD is the same as NAD in that it is capable of reversible oxidation and reduction. Hence FAD is also a carrier of electrons and hydrogens. This function of FAD is expressed not only in certain flavoenzyme reactions but also in the mitochondria where it acts as a component of the electron transport chain, and (like NAD) harnesses energy in the form of ATP. In fact, NAD and FAD working together produce twice the amount of ATP. The reduced forms of FMN and FAD are written as $FMNH_2$ and $FADH_2$, respectively.

- The FMN form of riboflavin is also found as a component of the electron transport chain in the mitochondria.

- Both FMN and FAD are also present in the liver microsomes where they serve as electron carriers in a similar fashion to their roles in the mitochondria. However, in the microsomes they serve primarily to hydroxylate various drugs including steroids.

- Through its coenzyme forms, riboflavin participates in all aspects of metabolism. It promotes the utilisation of various carbohydrate, fatty acid and amino acid substrates and enables energy production to ensure adequate maintenance of body tissues in adults and growth in children.

- The FMN form of the vitamin may have some stimulatory action on the incorporation of iodide into thyroglobulin in the thyroid gland.

- The conversion of riboflavin into FAD and FMN is impaired in hypothyroidism and adrenal insufficiency.

- Superficially, riboflavin may help maintain healthy skin and hair.

- Riboflavin may protect against some of the effects of chronic alcohol abuse.

Requirement

The average intake of riboflavin in typical Western diets is around 2 - 3 mg per day. Some 40 percent of our riboflavin requirement comes from milk and its products, another 20 percent comes from meats, and 15 percent is provided by various grain products. Eggs are also a good source of riboflavin. Further details are given in the compendium (Table 51.2).

People who are very active physically may have a slightly increased riboflavin requirement because of its extensive involvement in metabolic processes. Not all nutritionists agree that extra riboflavin is required by people who engage in above average activity. There is an increased requirement for riboflavin during pregnancy and lactation. Small amounts of riboflavin are found in the liver and kidneys, but excess riboflavin is rapidly excreted in the urine. It is believed that riboflavin may be synthesised by the gut bacteria in response to complex carbohydrates in the diet, and that some of this riboflavin may become available by absorption. The recommended adult daily intake of riboflavin in males is 13 mg/d and in females is 11 mg/d, respectively.

Toxicity

There is no known toxicity due to riboflavin. Up to 20 mg riboflavin may be taken over long periods with no side effects other than a harmless deep yellow coloration of the urine. However, an imbalance of other B-group vitamins may develop with prolonged use of riboflavin supplements on their own. High doses of riboflavin have been used to treat mouth ulcers in some patients. Other types of ulcers may also respond to such treatment for example corneal ulcers. Even doses as high as 100 to 200 mg have produced no side effects in the short term. Riboflavin is deemed so safe that it is permitted as a food colorant.

Deficiency

A deficiency of riboflavin is termed ariboflavinosis. Riboflavin deficiency on its own is rare in humans. Occasionally, however, it is seen as a complication of other vitamin deficiency diseases such as pellagra and beriberi. It may also accompany protein-energy malnutrition. Alcoholism or faddish diets may contribute to riboflavin deficiency. Elevated homocysteine levels can be associated with riboflavin deficiency. The humans, symptoms of riboflavin deficiency include cheilosis (cheilitis), a painful inflammation and cracking of the corners of the mouth, an oily dermatitis, a sore red tongue and throat, and vascularisation of the cornea of the eyes. A niacin deficiency has somewhat similar effects that make it difficult to distinguish from a pure riboflavin deficiency. In chronic cases of riboflavin deficiency, one of the most serious effects is progressive damage to the eyes. Conjunctivitis may develop which causes a burning sensation and a feeling of sandy grit in the eyes. The eyes may appear bloodshot and watery, and vision may be affected in both very bright and very dim light. The pupils may become dilated and ultimately vascularisation of the cornea and very often cataracts may develop.

The earlier and less serious condition called cheilosis is characterised by cracked lips especially at the corners of the mouth. Sore lines may also develop around the sides of the nose and a scaling of the skin on the lips, nose, forehead and ears may occur. The scalp may be affected and in severe cases hair loss may be evident. Acne or eczema may also develop which is occasionally accompanied by more generalised dermatitis around the body.

Some nervous symptoms occasionally occur such as shaking, dizziness and insomnia. A general muscular weakness may also develop. Some genital lesions may develop in severe cases. Although frank mental depression rarely occurs. Liver metabolism may be affected resulting in a fatty liver. A form of anaemia sometimes develops as a consequence of riboflavin deficiency which is characterised by a diminished production of otherwise normal red blood cells (sometimes referred to as normochromic normocytic anaemia). In part, this could be due to some induced defect in folate metabolism. Infants treated with phototherapy can develop riboflavin deficiency because of the light-sensitive nature of riboflavin. A riboflavin deficiency before birth may cause defects in the developing foetus. Riboflavin deficiency in young animals results in a failure to grow.

A group of volunteers who were maintained on a level of 0.5 mg riboflavin per day developed symptoms of cheilosis after about 120 days. It may be assumed that this condition would have developed even earlier in persons completely deprived of riboflavin. The generally accepted onset time is in the range 100 to 130 days. Patients with severe ariboflavinosis recover within a month when given supplements of around 5 mg riboflavin per day.

Table 52.1. Relative biopotency of different forms and
derivatives of riboflavin

NAME	NOMINAL VALUE (percent)
Riboflavin	100
Flavin mononucleotide (FMN)	80
Flavin dinucleotide (FAD)	50
Lumiflavin	0
Lumichrome	0

Because of their larger size, the coenzymes of riboflavin have relatively lower biopotencies. Theoretical values for FMN and FAD are approximately 80 and 50 percent respectively, on the above scale.

About 1 to 2 percent of the riboflavin in the body occurs as free riboflavin, up to 30 percent occurs as FMN, and 70 percent or more (occasionally 90 percent) occurs as FAD.

Table 52.2. Riboflavin compendium

FOOD GROUP	RIBOFLAVIN LEVEL
Milk and products	Medium
Eggs	High
Meat and fish	Very variable
Fats and oils	Nil
Grain and products	Medium
Nuts and pulses	Medium
Root vegetables	Low
Leaf vegetables	Medium
Fruit	Low
Sweets	Very low, variable

53

Thiamine

Common names

Thiamine.
Vitamin B_1.

Alternative Names

Thiamin. Aneurine. Aneurin. Oryzamin.
Torulin. Polyneuramin.
B_1. Part of B_{10}. Part of B_{11}. Vitamin F.
Antiberiberi factor (or activity).
Antineuritic factor (or vitamin).
Energy Vitamin.

Some of the above terms are obsolete or trivial.

History

-----: For centuries, the Chinese knew that tea made from rice bran was a cure for beriberi.

1881: Lunin showed that rats could not survive on a diet of carbohydrate, lipid, protein and minerals only.

1887: Takati prevented beriberi by reducing milled rice and increasing rations of milk, meat and vegetables for Japanese sailors.

1893: Eijkman produced paralysis in chickens by feeding them white rice.

1900: With Grijns, Eijkman cured this by feeding rice bran.

1906: Hopkins showed that some accessory food factors were necessary in the diet. His full paper was not published until 1912, when he announced that some factors in milk were essential for normal growth in animals.

1912: By 1912, Funk established that beriberi is caused by the lack of a specific chemical substance which he showed to be an amine. He formulated a theory of deficiency diseases called the vitamin theory, and coined the term Vitamine.

1915: McCollum and Davis distinguish between two growth factors in rats, namely fat-soluble A and water-soluble B. Only factor B cured beriberi.

1925: The term Vitamin B is considered to be a complex of more than one component.

1926: Jansen and Donath isolated a small quantity of Vitamin B_1.

1932: Windaus discovered that Vitamin B_1 contains a sulphur atom.

1936: Williams and Cline synthesised Vitamin B_1 and proposed the name Thiamine (also spelt Thiamin).

1937: Lohmann and Schuster isolated the heat-stable coenzyme (previously named cocarboxylase by Auhagen), involved with the enzyme pyruvate decarboxylase in yeast, and showed that it contained Thiamine in the form of Thiamine Pyrophosphate (TPP).

1952: Thiamine triphosphate was discovered in rat liver by Rossi-Fanelli et al.

Nature

Thiamine is synthesised by higher plants and most microorganisms, but is not available from the gut bacteria. There is only one natural form of thiamine, although many synthetic derivatives have been intensively studied in recent years. Chemically, thiamine consists of two ring structures linked by a methylene ($-CH_2-$) bridge. One of these rings is a substituted pyrimidine and the other is a substituted thiazole. Mild oxidants convert thiamine to the inactive breakdown product called thiochrome. Thiamine is a very unstable vitamin. The biopotencies of different forms of thiamine are given in Table 53.1. Pure thiamine carries one positive charge on its thiazole nitrogen.

This form may exist in solution, however in the solid form thiamine exists as a salt. The most common salt is the chloride. This contains additional Cl⁻ and HCl moieties in a crystalline structure.

Thiamine is a component of the coenzyme thiamine pyrophosphate (TPP, previously termed cocarboxylase). Chemically, the term pyrophosphate indicates a double phosphate or a diphosphate. The coenzyme therefore consists of thiamine linked to two phosphate groups (at the thiazole end).

TPP is involved as a coenzyme for several enzymes.

- The pyruvate dehydrogenase complex requires TPP to decarboxylate pyruvate giving acetyl-CoA. Acetyl-CoA is involved in cellular respiration in the citric acid cycle.

- The α-ketoglutarate dehydrogenase complex is another enzyme that requires TPP and is involved in the citric acid cycle in the matrix of the mitochondrion.

- The pyruvate decarboxylase complex (alpha-ketoacid carboxylase) catalyses the decarboxylation of pyruvic acid in the cytoplasm and mitochondria of animal cells.

- Branched-chain α-ketoacid dehydrogenase complex is an enzyme system located on the inner membrane of mitochondria. The complex catalyzes the oxidative decarboxylation of branched, short-chain α-ketoacids.

- Transketolase, occurring in the cytosol, is involved in the pentose phosphate pathway in all organisms.

- 2-Hydroxyphytanoyl-CoA lyase is an enzyme found in the peroxisome organelle and is involved in the oxidation of phytanoic acid.

Biological Functions

- Apart from free thiamine, the vitamin occurs in several phosphorylated forms, including thiamin monophosphate (TMP), thiamine diphosphate or thiamine pyrophosphate (TPP), and thiamin triphosphate (TTP).

• Thiamine monophosphate, TMP, has no known function other than being an intermediate in TPP and TTP synthesis and both are present in the diet.

• Thiamine pyrophosphate, TPP, is essential for two major types of reaction in the body, namely oxidative decarboxylation and transketolation. In both reactions, an activated aldehyde group (– CHO) is involved. Both decarboxylase and transketolase require TPP as a coenzyme and are components of larger multienzyme complexes in the cell. These complexes act on various α–keto acids such as pyruvate and α–ketoglutarate which are essential intermediates in carbohydrate metabolism.

• During reactions involving TPP, active aldehyde groups are formed. If the reaction is a decarboxylase, the aldehyde moiety is transferred to form acetyl-CoA in a process that also involves lipoic acid (see Chapter 63). On the other hand, if the reaction is a transketolase, the aldehyde moiety is transferred to various carbohydrate units to form larger carbohydrate units. The decarboxylase system occurs in the mitochondria of all cells in the body, whereas the transketolase system occurs mainly in the liver, adipose tissue and lactating mammary gland, where it occurs in the cytoplasm of the cell and not in the mitochondria.

• Through its role as a component of TPP, thiamine is essential to the metabolism of carbohydrates and, working together with CoA, it helps in the provision of acetate for synthesis of fatty acids, and also energy for the cell.

• Apart from fueling the citric acid cycle, the catabolism of the three branched chain amino acids, leucine, isoleucine, and valine, also contributes to the production of cholesterol and acts as a source of nitrogen for the synthesis of the neurotransmitters, glutamate and γ-aminobutyric acid.

• Thiamine has a role in maintaining the integrity of the nervous system. It is uniformly distributed throughout the nervous system and is localized in membrane structures. In this regard, it may assist in the mental process of learning and may help maintain a positive mental attitude. It also helps by preventing the irritability and depression which may occur in its absence.

- Thiamine triphosphate, TTP, may be an activator of chloride ion channels.

- Nerve stimulation results in a decline of the level of TTP and TPP in experimental preparations and in the release of TMP and free thiamine.

- Thiamine may protect against the effects of over-eating, by assisting in the digestion and assimilation of food. It also helps maintain good muscle tone in the gut. Also, one of its roles in this regard is the maintenance of a normal appetite

- Thiamine deficiency and decreased thiamine-dependent enzyme activity have been associated with Alzheimer's disease.
- Thiamine may help to protect against some of the effects of chronic alcohol abuse.

Requirement

Some 40 percent of our thiamine requirement is provided by grain products, another 20 percent comas from vegetables and a further 15 percent comes from various meats. In countries like Ireland, potatoes contribute up to 15 percent of the daily intake of thiamine. People living in many parts of the world, including certain groups in Western countries, are deficient in thiamine.

The requirement for thiamine is believed by most nutritionists to be related to carbohydrate intake, or more conveniently to energy expenditure, because of its extensive involvement in metabolic processes. The recommended adult daily intake of thiamine in males is 12 mg/d and in females is 11 mg/d, respectively.

It is worth noting that the energy content of human milk averages some 2,700 kJ per day, with a variation ranging from 1,500 to 4,200 kJ par day. During lactation, up to 0.2 mg thiamine may be secreted in the milk per day. When the additional energy content and vitamin content of the milk is considered, an additional thiamine allowance is generally recommended during lactation. An additional thiamine allowance is also recommended during pregnancy.

Toxicity

Oral thiamine is non-toxic. For example, doses as high as 200 mg thiamine can be taken without side effects. But continued use of supplements may cause an imbalance of other B-group vitamins. Part of the reason why thiamine is non-toxic is the fact that thiamine absorption from the gut is limited. About 15 mg per day appears to be the maximum dose the can be absorbed on high thiamine intakes. Another reason is the fact that excess thiamine is rapidly eliminated in the urine. On the other hand, hypersensitivity reactions may occur on high therapeutic (intravenous) doses of the vitamin. Symptoms of thiamine toxicity may include increased pulse rate with possibly irregular heart beat and low blood pressure, weakness, irritability, headache and insomnia.

Deficiency

Several factors deplete the thiamine reserves in the body such as smoking, drinking alcohol and excessive intake of carbohydrates. The eating of large amounts of certain types of raw fish and shellfish (including oysters) may also cause a deficiency of thiamine. This is because some raw fish contains a thiamine splitting enzyme called thiaminease. This enzyme is destroyed on cooking, and therefore there is no such risk on eating cooked fish.

The activity of the enzyme pyruvate decarboxylase decreases during thiamine deficiency. The activity of transketolase in the red blood cell also decreases. A consequence of these enzyme deficiencies is an increase in certain metabolites such as pyruvate, pentose sugars and □-keto derivatives of the amino acids leucine, isoleucine and valine. The buildup of pyruvate may sometimes cause laboured breathing. Although this symptom is more usually associated with haemorrhage into the ventricles of the brain in severe cases. The pyruvate also causes membranes to become more permeable causing oedema and dilation of small blood vessels. Constipation and abdominal cramps are also common in thiamine deficiencies. In a rare defect, the enzyme pyruvate decarboxylase tends to be inactive, and unless high doses of thiamine are administered there occurs a buildup of alanine. Similarly, another enzyme found in the liver, pyruvate carboxylase, may be defective and lead to a buildup of lactic acid unless high doses of the vitamin are administered.

Wernicke encephalopathy and Korsakoff syndrome are different conditions that often occur together. Wernicke-Korsakoff syndrome is a brain disorder due to thiamine deficiency. Early signs of thiamine deficiency include various nervous symptoms including irritability, apathy, lack of appetite, fatigue, weakness, poor learning and memory, and mental depression. Transketolase activity in the red blood cell decreases rapidly in thiamine deficiency. As the disease progresses, peripheral neuropathy occurs characterised by a feeling of pins and needles, or burning sensation in the extremities, starting with the toes and spreading upwards and eventually progressing to the hands. In extreme cases, Wernicke's syndrome (encephalopathy) may develop causing double vision, confusion, torpor, stupor, hallucinations and eventually coma and death. Some of these symptoms may also occur in severe alcoholism.

The symptoms of peripheral neuropathy (described above), often accompanied by paralysis, and muscle wasting are referred to as dry beriberi. In contrast, wet beriberi is characterised by heart damage. The heart muscle may be damaged and the heart may become enlarged and localised oedema may develop. The lining, of the heart and lungs may become inflamed and ultimately congestive heart failure accompanied by irregular heartbeats may develop. Sometimes a mixture of wet and dry beriberi symptoms may be present. Weight loss may occur in adults and the growth of children may be retarded. Some of the earliest symptoms such as nausea may occur within a week of thiamine deprivation. Personality changes accompanied by anxiety and confusion also occur early on in the course of the disease. The symptoms of beriberi (most notably those of wet beriberi) literally disappear overnight when thiamine is administered. The recovery is accompanied by a massive diuresis as the oedema recedes. Recently a superior form of thiamine called thiamine propyl disulfide has been used to treat cases of thiamine deficiency. Unlike the natural vitamin, the new form is not rate-limited by the absorption barrier in the gut. Of course, thiamine itself will work as well, but may take longer because during malnutrition (including alcoholism) the rate of absorption of thiamine may be even more limited than normal. Ruminants such as cattle, sheep and goats do not suffer from thiamine deficiencies as their gut bacteria provide their full requirement.

A third type of beriberi, infantile beriberi, occurs in very young children whose mothers have an inadequate thiamine intake. This condition rapidly leads to death unless the deficiency is corrected.

The order of development of thiamine deficiency symptoms has been studied in detail in a group of people on very low (0.2 mg per day) intakes. Urinary excretion of thiamine decreases progressively, averaging 50 μg (per day) after 5 days, 25 μg after 10 days, 10 μg after 25 days, and becomes negligible after about 100 days. The transketolase activity of the red blood cells progressively decreases after about 10 days, becoming 20 percent lower after 25 days, 35 percent lower after 100 days, and 50 percent lower after about 200 days. Loss of weight, irritability and insomnia commence after about 20 days, progressive weakness, polyneuritis, oedema, slow pulse and eye problems are evident after about 100 days. Enlargement of the heart and pathology of the cellular structures resulting from biochemical lesions begin to occur after about 200 days. These symptoms would develop at a somewhat faster rate in the complete absence of dietary thiamine.

Table 53.1. Relative biopotency of different forms
of thiamine

NAME	NOMINAL VALUE (percent)
Thiamine hydrochloride	100
Thiamine mononitrate	103
Thiamine pyrophosphate	80
Thiochrome	0

Thiamine hydrochloride and thiamine mononitrate are the most common supplementary forms of the vitamin. Because of its larger size, the coenzyme thiamine pyrophosphate has a lower biopotency which is theoretically about 80 percent on the above scale.

Table 53.2. Thiamine compendium

FOOD GROUP	THIAMINE LEVEL
Milk and products	Very low
Eggs	Low
Meat / Fish	Medium, variable / Low
Fats and oils	Nil
Grain and products	High
Nuts and pulses	High, variable
Root vegetables	Very low
Leaf vegetables	Low
Fruit	Low, variable
Sweets	Very low, variable

54

Folate

Common names

Folate.
Folic Acid.
Vitamin B$_9$.

Alternative Names

Norit eluate factor. Wills factor.
Antianaemia vitamin (or factor).
Factor U, Factor H, Factor R, T component.
Citrovorum Factor. Folic acid group. Foliage factor.
Vitamin B$_c$. Vitamin R. Vitamin M.
Vitamin B$_9$. Vitamin B$_{10}$. Vitamin B$_{11}$.
Pteroyl-L-glutamic acid. PGA.
Pteroyl-(n)-glutamates.
Pteroyl-oligo-γ–glutamates.
Lactobacillus cassei factor.
SLR factor. Fermentation factor.
5-formyl tetrahydrofolate.
Folacin. Folinic Acid.
Levomefolic acid, L-methylfolate, 5-MTHF.

Many of the above terms are obsolete.

History

-----: A tropical form of anaemia (Sprue) was known in India and elsewhere for many years.

1885: Work by Hopkins on flavins in butterfly wings anticipated the importance of folic acid and related chemicals.

1931: Wills discovered that a form of macrocytic anaemia in humans could be cured by certain liver and yeast extracts.

1938: Day discovered that yeast cured a nutritional blood disorder in monkeys which could be induced by feeding the local Indian diet.

1939: Hogan and Parrot showed that a similar anaemia in chickens could be prevented using liver extracts.

1940: A growth factor for certain bacteria was isolated from liver by Snell and Peterson. In the following year, Hutchings found that this factor was essential for chickens.

1941: Mitchell, *at al.*, isolated a similar growth factor from spinach which is named folic acid (foliage factor). By this time, it was realised that factors from numerous sources such as liver, yeast, alfalfa and spinach all have a chemical structure in common.

1943: Stockad showed that there are several different forms of folic acid containing glutamic acid residues. Hence the alternative name pteroylglutamic acid (PGA).

1945: Spies demonstrated that folic acid also cured anaemia in humans.

1946: Angier, *et al.*, were the first to isolate, characterise and synthesise pteroylglutamic acid.

1949: The Citrovorum Factor (a bacterial growth factor) was discovered. This active coenzyme form of the vitamin was shown to be N^5formyltetrahydrofolic acid (Folinic Acid). Folinic Acid has also been known as CoF. Several derivatives of folic acid are now known to be biologically active coenzymes involved in one carbon metabolism.

circa 1970: It became clear that the natural poly–γ–glutamyl side chain derivatives of folic acid are the preferred coenzymes for enzymes and are often more active and better retained in the cell.

-----: Folate is now a generic term for all natural derivatives of folic acid which exhibit qualitatively the biological activity of folic acid itself. Folic acid may occur with from one to nine glutamic acid residues, and the term folinic acid includes the reduced forms bearing various one-carbon moieties. Over 150 forms of folate have been reported. The measure, Dietary Folate Equivalents (DFE) includes the contribution of natural folates and synthetic folic acid (if present) to the total vitamin activity.

Nature

Folate is synthesised by higher plants and microorganisms. Folate also occurs in animal tissues where it is derived from plant sources. The structure of folate as extracted from plant, animal and bacteria differs according to the number of glutamic acid (glutamate) residues present. The term folate can be used as a generic descriptor for all natural derivatives with folic acid activity. Folic acid consists chemically of three different types of units. A substituted pteridine double ringed structure is first linked directly to *para*-aminobenzoic acid forming the basic pteroic acid structure. This in turn may be linked to glutamic acid residues, the number of which can vary according to the source of the vitamin. When there is only one glutamate residue present the compound is called pteroylmonoglutamic acid or simply folic acid (strictly free folic acid).

All the natural polyglutamate forms are found in the γ–glutamyl linkage. The commoner proteolytic enzymes are not very effective with γ–linkages. Therefore, in the intestines the polyglutamic acids are hydrolysed by specific enzymes to release the free folic acid and various glutamic acid residues. The most common form of folate produced by bacteria contains three glutamate residues. The most common storage form in the liver in animals contains five glutamate residues. And the most common form found in higher plants contains seven glutamate residues. In general, the longer the side chain of glutamate residues the lower is the relative biopotency of the folate. The biopotencies of several forms of folate are given in Table 54.1, for convenience.

The *para*-aminobenzoic acid residue itself has no folate activity in humans, although in plants and microorganisms it may be used to synthesise the vitamin. There is a possibility that some gut bacteria, in particular, the probiotic, *Lactobacillus plantarum*, may be able to provide some folic acid from dietary *para*-aminobenzoate. But the extent of this contribution is uncertain. Folate is a very unstable vitamin. A large number of folic acid derivatives occur in nature and many more have been synthesised.

Folic acid is a component of a group of coenzymes derived from tetrahydrofolic acid, THFA. These coenzymes consist of the basic folic acid structure of a pteridine linked to *para*-aminobenzoic acid which in turn is linked to one or more glutamic acid residues. However, four additional hydrogen atoms have been added to one of the pteridine rings thus reducing it to form the 5,6,7,8-tetrahydrofolic acid parent compound. Like the storage forms of folic acid, its coenzymes may also contain from one to several glutamate residues linked in γ–glutamyl linkage. These conjugates are of uncertain significance at the present time, although it appears that they are better retained by certain enzymes hence have prolonged activity in the cell.

Folate and folic acid are often used as synonymous terms by different authors. But in nutrition and dietetics there is an important distinction between the use of the two terms. Folates are relatively unstable tetrahydrofolate (polyglutamate) derivatives occurring naturally in foods. Folic acid is pteroylmonoglutamic acid (pteroyl-L-glutamate), a fully oxidized stable synthetic analog, used in food fortification and in supplements. This form of folic acid is not significantly found in foods. Natural folates are metabolized to 5-methyltetrahydrofolic acid (5-MTHF) in the mucosa of the small intestine. In contrast, synthetic folic acid is reduced and methylated in the liver. Subsequent conversion to the tetrahydrofolate form requires dihydrofolate reductase, an enzyme which is unusually slow in humans.

The term Dietary Folate Equivalent (DFE) includes the contribution of all vitamers to folate activity. Dietary Folate Equivalents depend on vitamer sources and circumstances. About 50% of folate naturally present in food is bioavailable, whereas at least 85% of synthetic folic acid is bioavailable when taken with food. The following shows the amount in μg giving one μg DFE under different conditions.

Natural folates derived from unfortified food   1.0

Folic acid derived from fortified food   0.6
or supplements taken with food

Folic acid derived from supplements   0.5
taken on an empty stomach

To calculate the DFE of a fortified food, it is necessary to know the micrograms of natural folate and synthetic folic acid present.

Biological Functions

- Around 10 - 19 mg of folate may be stored in the human body. Half of this occurs in the liver.

- All functions of folate are performed by tetrahydrofolate and its one-carbon derivatives. Irrespective of the number of glutamate residues, all the coenzyme forms are involved in one-carbon metabolism. Some textbooks consider THFA as a single coenzyme and its various one-carbon derivatives simply as reaction intermediates. Other authors take the view that each derivative may be considered as a distinct coenzyme. Suffice it to say that THFA serves as a carrier for (or donor of) a variety of one-carbon units including formyl (–CHO), hydroxymethyl (–CH_2OH), methyl (–CH_3), methylene (=CH_2), methenyl (=CH–), and formimino (–CH=NH) groups. Occasionally, the one-carbon units are classified according to their level of oxidation. These fall into three groups, namely the methyl (–CH_3) level, the aldehyde (O=CH_2) level which includes the methylene bridge, and the formyl (O=CH–) level which includes all the other derivatives.

- These one-carbon groups are involved in the synthesis of a large variety of compounds in the body. They may become attached to the number 5 nitrogen, N^5, or the number 10 nitrogen, N^{10}, of the basic coenzyme structure, and all are metabolically interconvertible in the body, thanks to the presence of no less than a dozen specific enzymes. The amino acid serine is the principle supplier of one-carbon units in the form of hydroxymethyl groups. The enzyme serine transhydroxymethylase found equally in the mitochondria and the cytoplasm catalyses the reaction. After becoming attached, these groups are unstable and rapidly convert to methylene bridges. Histidine is another source of carbon in the form of formimino groups ($-CH=NH_2$). These groups are in turn converted to methenyl bridges. In the red blood cell, formic acid may also contribute such carbon moieties to THFA. Table 54.2 lists the various one-carbon derivatives of THFA that act as interconvertible coenzymes in the body.

- Methylene-THFA is involved in the synthesis of methionine and other molecules such as choline, sarcosine and dimethylglycine. The coenzyme is first reduced to methyl-THFA and the new methyl group is transferred directly to the relevant substrate. In turn the methyl group received by methionine can be further transferred to synthesise other molecules in the cell.

- Methylene-THFA may also add a hydroxymethyl group to glycine to form serine (which is the reverse of the normal reaction providing carbon moieties to THFA).

- Methylene-THFA is also involved in the formation of the pyrimidine nucleoside containing thymine, in the presence of an enzyme called thymidylate synthetase. The overall result of this reaction is the addition of a methyl group to the number 5 carbon of a uracil derivative. Hydrogens are also transferred in this complex reaction resulting in 6,7-dihydrofolic acid as an intermediate coenzyme form. Thymine is one of the pyrimidine bases (together with cytosine and uracil) which is required in nucleic acid synthesis. The thymine synthesising enzyme is inhibited by methotrexate which is a powerful drug used as an anticancer agent. Methotrexate displaces the folic acid coenzyme from the enzyme, thus inactivating it. In the absence of thymine, DNA cannot be synthesised and cells cannot continue to grow. Many cancer cells die within 36 hours. After treatment with methotrexate type drugs, cancer patients may be rescued by administering folinic acid.

- Both methenyl- and N^{10}-formyl- THFA are required for the synthesis of the purine nucleotide called inosine-5-phosphate. The methylene carbon is incorporated as the number 8 carbon in the purine ring structure. And the formyl carbon is incorporated as the number 2 carbon in the presence of tranformylase enzymes. Inosine may be further converted to other purine nucleosides containing adenine and guanine which are essential also in the synthesis of nucleic acids.

- Methyl-THFA is involved in the transfer of methyl groups to cobalamin to form methylcobalamin, one of the vitamin B_{12} coenzymes. This reaction is considered again in Chapter 56.

- Folinic aid is very stable form of THFA that can be administered orally to provide reduced folate not requiring the activity of the enzyme called dihydrofolate reductase. Normally after free folic acid is absorbed it must be reduced by this enzyme to form THFA. Folinic acid is converted directly to methyl-THFA during absorption in the intestine.

- Tetrahydrobiopterin helps to oxidise the amino acid phenylalanine to tyrosine.

- Through its metabolic reactions as outlined above, folate is widely involved in synthetic reactions involving amino acids and nucleic acid bases. Through these actions, folate ensures proper growth and development of cells and the transmission of genetic information. Folate maintains the integrity of the genome. It ensures adequate DNA synthesis, RNA synthesis and protein synthesis. And in particular, it is essential for the maturation of liver cells and red blood cells.

- Folate also helps the appetite and stimulates the production of hydrochloric acid in the stomach.

- Folate may help to improve lactation in certain cases.

- It has been claimed but not proven that folate together with pantothenic acid and *para*-aminobenzoic acid may offset premature greying of hair and promote a healthy complexion.

• Folate may be of therapeutic value in certain cases of schizophrenia.

• Folate may also be of therapeutic value in the treatment of stomach and leg ulcers, glossitis (sore tongue), and circulation particularly in arthritic patients.

• Folate protects against the effects of free radicals and oxidation.

• Folate may help to counteract some of the effects of chronic alcohol abuse.

Requirement

Folate is not well absorbed from the gut. Up to about one-half of the total folate in some diets may be in the free folic acid form. This is the readily available form. In other diets, the free component may be nearer one-quarter of the total. Polyglutamates of folic acid must first be hydrolysed before the folic acid component can be absorbed. The best sources of folate include yeast, grain products, vegetables, liver, kidney and milk. A compendium gives further details on total folate content of various foods (Table 54.3).

The bioavailability of folate in various foods is variable. In general, it is useful to consider the following values which have been established. The average free folic acid content (as a percentage of the total folate) of various food groups is as follows: milk, 80; eggs, 55; kidneys, 80; other meats 55; fish, 30; grain products, 25 - 50; nuts and pulses, 25; root vegetables, 75; leaf vegetables 80 - 90; and fruit, 50 - 55, percent, respectively.

As a rule, most of the free folic acid is absorbed, however much of this is rapidly lost again in the urine. Small amounts of the diglutamic acid form of folate may also be absorbed. But the percentage of the total folate in individual foods which is absorbed is not yet known with certainty. In the meantime, recommended intakes are usually based on the assumption that on average only 25 percent of the total folate in the diet will be absorbed. When fully saturated, the body may contain up to 20 mg folate.

A minimum amount of free folic acid, corresponding to about 50 µg per day, is necessary to prevent anaemia and maintain folate balance in the body. However, as much as 200 µg of free folic acid is necessary per day to restore normal blood plasma levels in anaemic patients. Currently, the recommended adult daily intake of folate in both males and females is 400 µg/d. These daily intakes should ensure adequate folate status of the liver. Additional folate supplementation is recommended to maintain normal red blood cell folate levels in pregnant women. The recommended folate intake during pregnancy is one and a half times the normal adult value for women. The folate content of breast milk is around 80 µg per litre. So, additional folate is also recommended during lactation.

The requirement for folate is also increased during hyperthyroidism and haemolytic anaemia. In general, it is believed that there is an increased requirement for folate whenever the rate of one-carbon metabolism is increased in the body. However, no values for this have been set to date. The average intake of folate in the typical Western diet is around 150 to 250 µg per day. In some countries, the average intake can be as low as 50 mg per day. However, with diets rich in vegetables, the intake may be as high as 2,000 µg per day.

Toxicity

Folate is relatively non-toxic because excess is rapidly excreted in the urine. Excessive intake may however cause imbalance of other B-group vitamins. Also, there is a risk that high intakes of folate may mask some symptoms of a vitamin B_{12} deficiency. This is serious, because although the blood picture may be corrected, the underlying cause of the deficiency is not, and may lead to the more serious neurological disorders which are associated with chronic vitamin B_{12} deficiency. If folate intake exceeds 15 mg per day, direct toxic symptoms may develop. These include nausea, diarrhoea, flatulence, bloat, irritability and loss of appetite. Also, the sleep patterns may be disturbed. In general, it is not recommended to take more than 500 µg folate as a supplement per day. This is because 300 to 500 µg is sufficient to correct anaemia if it is due to folate deficiency, but it is not enough to mask a vitamin B_{12} deficiency.

Deficiency

Folate deficiency is the most common vitamin deficiency in developed countries. There is a risk of folate deficiency in human diets, particularly those lacking in vegetables. Sprue is a deficiency disease of uncertain origin but is frequently associated with folate deficiency. It is characterised by impaired absorption of a number of nutrients, including lipids leading to steatorrhoea (fatty faeces), diarrhoea, weight loss, skin pigmentation, megaloblastic arrest of the bone marrow, and ultimately macrocytic anaemia. Deficiency of folate results in blood disorders including anaemia and decreased white blood cells. Anaemia resulting from folate deficiency is characterised by a reduced number of larger than normal (often malformed) red blood cells which usually contain a normal complement of haemoglobin. This condition is sometimes termed megaloblastic, or macrocytic, normochromic anaemia. The fundamental cause of this condition is believed to be the shortage of DNA that a folate (or indirectly a vitamin B_{12}) deficiency produces. The key intermediate in thymine synthesis, namely methylene-THFA, requires both folate and vitamin B_{12} for its formation. This view is supported by the evidence that administering high doses of thymine alone in some cases causes an improvement in the anaemia associated with sprue and also, occasionally, in pernicious anaemia. The anaemia associated with sprue responds dramatically to folate.

Similarly, macrocytic anaemias of pregnancy and infancy have a good response. It is believed that the underlying cause of these deficiency symptoms is a failure of DNA synthesis, which is required to direct haemoglobin production in the maturing red blood cell. Deficiency of folate during pregnancy may result in foetal damage. A serious folate deficiency problem includes neural tube defects. It is recommended that women planning to conceive, should take supplements of folate which can prevent 50 percent or more of neural tube defects such as spina bifida and anencephaly.

Deficiency in children results in retardation of growth. The ratio of DNA to RNA in a normal blood cell is just over 3 to 1. In folate deficiency, this ratio can decrease towards 1. The steatorrhoea may be due to atrophy of the small intestine particularly in the jejunum area where there is normally a very rapid replacement of the cells of the mucosa. Again, DNA is required to maintain this process.

The enzyme dihydrofolate reductase is required for the conversion of folic acid to THFA. This occurs in two steps. The first step yields 7,8-dihydrofolic acid and the second step completes the reaction to yield 5,6,7,8-tetrahydrofolic acid. The enzyme may be inhibited by drugs called antifolate agents. Such drugs may also act as competitive inhibitors of folate by displacing folate from the active sites of key enzymes, and they have been used to combat certain types of cancer including leukemia. The rationale here is the fact that folate coenzymes are required for the development of cancer cells and white blood cells in particular which are overproduced in leukemia. Therefore, inhibitors of coenzyme synthesis or competitive inhibitors of folate coenzymes may act by inhibiting excess white cell production. Immunosuppressant drugs such as aminopterin and methotrexate have had some success in prolonging life in such cases. Other drugs, particularly antibiotics such as trimetoprim and streptomycin inhibit the production of folate by the gut bacteria and may thus indirectly lead to folate deficiency. Vitamin C may also be involved in the reduction of folic acid to THFA and a serious deficiency of vitamin C may therefore sometimes lead to symptoms of folate deficiency. Rats and mice with folate deficiency develop a copious diarrhoea and bone marrow disorders. One test for folate deficiency is the accumulation of formiminoglutamic acid when a loading dose of the amino acid histidine is administered. Normally the formimino group is transferred to form the coenzyme formimino-THFA.

In a rare disorder of folic acid transport resulting in poor absorption of the vitamin, higher than normal doses of the vitamin may be required to offset deficiency symptoms. A decreased ability to ward off infections may be evident in some cases of folate deficiency, particularly in young infants. Other more general symptoms of folate deficiency include fatigue, irritability, insomnia and certain mental symptoms such as poor memory and confusion.

The development of folate deficiency has been studied in detail in the human. After about 10 days, serum levels of folic acid are noticeably decreased. After about 50 days there is excessive segmentation of the white blood cells called leucocytes. After about 100 days, formiminoglutamic acid appears in the urine. Also around that time there is a noticeably lower folic acid content in the red blood cells. Megaloblastic arrest of the bone marrow commences at around 120 days. And this leads on to the full blown macrocytic anaemia after about 150 days.

Table 54.1. Relative biopotency of different forms and derivatives
of folate

NAME	NUMBER OF GLUTAMATE RESIDUES	NOMINAL VALUE (percent)
Free folic acid	1	100
Bacterial folate	3	65
Animal folate	5	45
Plant folate	7	35
para-Aminobenzoic acid	0	0
Glutamic acid	1	0

The above values should be interpreted as theoretical optimum
biopotencies. The actual values would depend on the relative
bioavailability of different forms of folate in the diet. The various
coenzyme forms of folate are all approximately the same size (for
any fixed number of glutamate residues). Hence they all have
approximately the same biopotency, which is not significantly less
than the relative biopotency of their corresponding polyglutamate
form. The greatest difference would occur for the monoglutamate
forms and in that case the theoretical biopotency of the various
one-carbon derivatives is only 5 percent less than the value for free
folic acid. The possibility that some coenzyme forms may have a
greater activating effect on certain enzymes does not mean that
they are more potent in the sense used throughout (which refers to
oral doses). Whatever the final number of glutamate residues, the
coenzyme forms are all derived in the body from folic acid itself.

Table 54.2. Folic acid and coenzyme derivatives of
tetrahydrofolic acid

NAME LINKAGE	GROUP ATTACHED	POSITION
Folic acid	----	----
Dihydrofolic acid	----	----
Tetrahydrofolic acid (THFA)	----	----
Formyl-THFA (Folinic acid)	$-CHO$	N^5
Formyl-THFA	$-CHO$	N^{10}
Hydroxymethyl-THFA	$-CH_2OH$	N^{10}
Methyl-THFA	$-CH_3$	N^5
Methylene-THFA	$=CH_2$	N^5, N^{10}
Methenyl-THFA	$=CH-$	N^5, N^{10}
Formimino-THFA	$-CHNH_2$ $(-CH=NH)$ $(-CH=N^+H_2)$	N^5
Tetrathydrobiopterin (THB)	----	----

Folinic acid is a very stable form. Hydroxymethyl-THFA is an unstable
intermediate. Tetrahydrobiopterin is a cofactor which is related to folic
acid and also has some structure resemblances to riboflavin. Some
older terms for folinic acid were Coenzyme F, CoF, Citrovorum Factor
and Leucovorin. Occasionally, methenyl-THFA had been termed
Anhydrocitrovorum. These terms are no longer used. See text for
further details.

Table 54.3. Folate compendium

FOOD GROUP	FOLATE LEVEL
Milk and products	Low
Eggs	Low
Meat and fish	Very variable
Fats and oils	Nil
Grain and products	Medium, variable
Nuts and pulses	High
Root vegetables	Very low
Leaf vegetables	Medium, variable
Fruit	Very low, variable
Sweets	Nil

55

Biotin

Common names

Biotin.
Vitamin B$_7$.

Alternative names

D-Biotin. Biotin-d.
Protective Factor X. Vitamin H.
Bios II. Bios IIB. Coenzyme R (CoR). Factor X. Vitamin B$_w$.
Vitamin B$_4$. Factor S. Factor W.
Egg-white injury preventative factor. Anti-stress Vitamin. The Skin Vitamin.

Many of the above terms are obsolete.

History

1901: Wilders discovered that yeast required a substance in wort, called Bios, for growth (see also Pantothenic Acid, Chapter 50).

1916: The detrimental effect of feeding raw egg white to animals was first noticed by Bateman.

1927: Boas cured this 'egg white injury' with a factor found in liver which he called 'Protective Factor X.

circa 1930: A factor necessary for the growth of certain *Rhizobia* bacteria (hence called Coenzyme R), was discovered.

1931: Paul György, independently discovers a similar factor in liver and calls it Vitamin H.

1936: Kogl and Tonnis isolated and crystallised a pure substance from egg yolk which they called biotin, and in the following year they reported its structure.

1940: Paul György *et al.*, showed that biotin cured the deficiency of Vitamin H in animals (and was therefore the same compound). In the following year, du Vigneaud confirmed the structure. Factors from several sources including Bios were shown to be one and the same vitamin.

1945: Biotin was synthesised by Harris.

1963: Lynen confirmed (the original suggestion of Lardy, *et al.*) that biotin acts as a coenzyme (CoR), and showed that its structure contains lysine, in the form of Biocytin. The coenzyme is involved in carboxylations which are essential for a wide variety of metabolic reactions in the cell.

Nature

Biotin can be synthesised in higher plants and many microorganisms. In the human, biotin is a conditionally essential nutrient. A large portion of the biotin requirement in humans is supplied by the gut bacteria. There are eight isomers of biotin but D-biotin is the only biologically active form. Biotin consists of two fused rings one of which contains a sulphur atom. This ring also contains a short chain consisting of five carbon atoms, ending with a carboxyl (–COOH) group.

Three derivatives of biotin have been found in natural foods. These are biocytin which is probably a breakdown product of a biotin-protein complex, and the D- and L- sulfoxides of biotin. All three support the growth of some bacteria, but their efficacy as substitutes for biotin itself in human nutrition is not yet fully known. In biocytin, a lysine residue is attached to the short side chain resulting in a compound named epsilon-N-biotinyl-L-lysine (or ε–N-biotinyl-L-lysine). As stated above, it is believed to be a part of a protein complex called carboxybiotin enzyme. The sulphoxides of biotin contain an additional atom of oxygen linked to the sulphur atom. Thiamine is the only other vitamin known to contain a sulphur atom.

A number of other derivatives of biotin have been studied in recent years, but the results are as yet unclear as far a human nutrition is concerned. What is clear is the fact that biotin can be largely supplied by the gut bacteria in humans and it is difficult to produce deficiencies. The relative potencies of several forms of biotin are illustrated in Table 55.1. These values are only approximate and they are not completely certain at present. Biotinol differs from biotin only in the chain ending group which is an hydroxymethyl ($-CH_2OH$) instead of a carboxyl ($-COOH$). Oxybiotin contains an oxygen atom which is substituted for the sulphur atom. And dethiobiotin has lost the sulphur atom resulting in ring opening. Other analogues of biotin actually act as potent inhibitors of the vitamin function. Biotin is a relatively stable vitamin.

Biological Functions

• Biotin serves as a coenzyme when it is linked to various carboxylase enzymes through an amide linkage to the ε–amino group of a lysine residue. The coenzyme itself may be considered as the biotin-lysine unit called ε–N-biotiny-L-lysine, or biocytin for short (previously termed Coenzyme R or CoR). Biotin-dependent carboxylase enzymes include pyruvate carboxylase and acetyl-, propyl-, and β–methylcrotonyl-, CoA carboxylases. These enzymes are essential in carbohydrate and fatty acid metabolism. All these enzymes depend on one additional enzyme, called holocarboxylase synthetase, to link the biotin and lysine residues to form biocytin, the coenzyme that activates them.

• Not only is biotin involved in the conversion of substrates in intermediary metabolism, but it is also involved in the production of energy. Biotin, as a coenzyme, promotes the oxidation of carbohydrates and lipids, the synthesis of fatty acids and, in particular, the metabolism of polyunsaturated fatty acids. Biotin also assists in the deamination of several amino acids and the synthesis of citrulline in the kidney urea cycle.

• Biotin is essential to a process called the fixation of carbon dioxide, were molecules of CO_2 are incorporated into larger molecules in the body. The synthesis of purines is one example where this mechanism is essential. Hence the importance of biotin in nucleic acid synthesis.

• Biotin cooperates in the utilisation of other vitamins, particularly pantothenic acid, folate and vitamin B_{12}.

• Through its various metabolic functions biotin helps maintain the healthy condition of skin including the scalp, nervous tissue, bone marrow, gonads and the sweat glands.

• Biotin promotes healthy hair. It may slow down the development of premature baldness in some males, but in most cases, it has no effect on this condition.

• Biotin, along with other B-group vitamins, helps the body to cope with stress.

Requirement

Yeast, eggs, various meats, particularly liver, and peanuts are good sources of biotin. The compendium gives further details although it should be noted that the bioavailability of biotin from different sources varies greatly (Table 54.3). The recommended adult daily intake of biotin in both males and in females is 30 µg/d. Some researchers recommend that more biotin per day may be required on occasion, particularly during pregnancy and lactation. During pregnancy for example the blood levels of biotin are slightly lower than normal. However, it has been suggested that the gut bacteria in healthy people may be capable of providing all the biotin that they need. This conclusion is based on the observation that some 3 to 6 times more biotin than the amount provided in the diet alone is normally excreted in the urine per day.

Toxicity

There is no known toxicity due to biotin in humans. Even infants on 10 mg per day do not develop symptoms. Excess biotin is excreted by the kidneys in urine. However, excessive supplementation with biotin may lead to disturbances in the levels of other B-group vitamins in the body. In one report, excess biotin (10 mg) plus pantothenic acid (300 mg), taken for two months by an elderly woman, produced a case of eosinophilic pleuropericardial effusion.

Deficiency

A deficiency of biotin in humans is very rare. Egg white if taken regularly can induce biotin deficiency because the protein avidin combines with both dietary and gut bacterial biotin thus preventing absorption. Indeed, it is difficult to otherwise induce deficiencies even experimentally, although prolonged treatment with antibiotics may also contribute to biotin deficiencies in some cases. Infants occasionally develop biotin deficiency. First, infants do not have fully developed gut bacterial system, and second, human milk is normally very low in available biotin. This is why liver which is rich in biotin was often recommended for nursing mothers in the olden days.

The symptoms of biotin deficiency include greyish dry skin, dermatitis, hair loss, eczema and diarrhoea. Further symptoms include nervous irritability, stress, lack of appetite, lack of energy and muscular pains. A slight anaemia may develop. A number of mental symptoms including sleeplessness, apathy, and even depression, in severe cases, have occurred occasionally. Lipid metabolism may eventually be disturbed. A deficiency of the immune system may become evident in chronic cases. Low levels of biotin have been found in some infants who died of cot deaths, but the implications of these findings are not yet fully understood.

In a very rare disorder where biotin is present in the body but cannot become attached to carboxylase enzymes, symptoms of biotin deficiency may also occur. The reason for this condition is the absence of the special linking enzyme called holocarboxylase synthetase. If this enzyme is inactive then all the carboxylase enzymes cannot function properly and their substrates buildup in the body and eventually appear in the urine. These substrates include lactate, methylcrotonate, hydroxypropionate, and hydroxyisovalerate. A rare defect in the enzyme propionyl-CoA carboxylase itself, which leads to a buildup of propionic acid, may be corrected by administering large doses of biotin.

Fortunately, cooked eggs, unlike raw eggs, do not have the effect of preventing biotin absorption from the gut. This is because cooking causes a change in the protein (coagulation) which denatures the avidin. In one study, biotin deficiency was produced in a group of volunteers by depriving them of dietary biotin. It took about 70 days to produce symptoms of nausea, fatigue, sleepiness, depression and loss of weight. Some signs of neuropathy were also observed. However, there is some doubt about the interpretation of these findings and (as stated above) it has even been suggested that dietary sources of biotin may not be required in the diet

The sequence of events in the development of experimental biotin deficiency are as follows. After 20 to 30 days a scaly appearance of the skin develops which in some cases leads to dermatitis after only 50 days. At about 50 days the urinary excretion of biotin has decreased to 15 percent of its normal value. After 60 days, mild mental depression, fatigue, generalised muscle pains and dermatitis occur. And after 70 days, a lack of appetite, nausea, a slight anaemia, an increase in bile pigments, and a dramatic increase in blood cholesterol may be evident.

Table 55.1. Relative biopotencies of different forms of biotin

NAME	NOMINAL VALUE (percent)
D-Biotin	100
Biocytin	65
Biotinol	50, or less
Oxybiotin	30, or less
Biotin Sulfoxides	0
Bisnorbiotin	0
Dethiobiotin	0
Other isomers of Biotin	0

Because of its larger size, the coenzyme biocytin has a lower biopotency than D-biotin, and is theoretically around 65 percent on the above scale.

Table 55.2. Biotin compendium

FOOD GROUP	BIOTIN LEVEL
Milk and products	Low
Eggs	Very high
Meat and fish	Very variable
Fats and oils	Nil
Grain and products	Medium, variable
Nuts / Pulses	Very high / Medium, variable
Root vegetables	Very low
Leaf vegetables	Low, variable
Fruit	Very low
Sweets	Nil

56

Vitamin B_{12}

Common names

Vitamin B_{12}.
Cobalamin.

Alternative names

B_{12} Group. Corrinoids. Animal protein factor.
Zoopherin. Cow manure factor. Cyanobalamin. Cyanocobalamin.
Extrinsic factor. B_{12}. Anti-pernicious anaemia factor (or vitamin).
Vitamin T component. Nitrocobalamin.
Hydroxy-, adenosyl-, and methyl- cobalamin.
LLD *(Lactobacillus lactis* Dorner) factor.
Aquocobalamin (Aquacobalamin).
Hydroxocobalamin (Hydroxycobalamin).
Vitamin B_{12a}, B_{12b}, B_{12c}, 12a, 12b, 12c, 12r, 12s, 12III, V_{1a}.

Most of the above terms are obsolete.

History

1824: Combe attributed a case of pernicious anaemia to a disorder of the digestive system.

1849: Addison is the first to describe pernicious anaemia in detail.

1926: Minot and Murphy cured the disease with a liver diet.

1929: Castle showed that the absorption of the antipernicious anaemia factor (Extrinsic Factor) required another factor (Intrinsic Factor) found in the stomach lining.

1948: The cyanocobalamin form of Vitamin B_{12} was isolated concurrently by Rickes, *et al.*, and by Smith, *et al.* The vitamin was crystallised and named Vitamin B_{12} by Smith and Parker. West demonstrated the clinical activity of Vitamin B_{12} in relieving pernicious anaemia in humans.

1950: The hydroxocobalamin form of the vitamin was discovered. It had identical activity to the cyano- form which was subsequently found to be an artifact.

1955: Hodgkin determined the complete structure of Vitamin B_{12} which is the only vitamin to contain a metal atom, namely cobalt. (She received Nobel Prize in chemistry in 1964.)

1958: Coenzyme forms of Vitamin B_{12} were isolated by Barker *et al.*, and concurrently by Weissbach, *et al.*

1961: The structure of this coenzyme was determined, and Vitamin B_{12} was shown to be a component linked with either a methyl- or an adenosyl- moiety.

1972: The total synthesis of Vitamin B_{12} was accomplished by collaborating research groups of Woodward and of Eschenmoser.

1974: According to Linnel, *et al.*, there are three natural forms of Vitamin B_{12} in humans, namely hydroxy-, adenosyl, and methyl-cobalamin, respectively.

-----: The term Vitamin B_{12} is now used as a generic descriptor for all corrinoids containing copper that exhibit qualitatively the biological activity of cyanocobalamin.

Nature

Vitamin B_{12} is not synthesised in higher plants or animals. Only microorganisms can synthesise vitamin B_{12}. The gut bacteria contribute a small amount to the vitamin requirement in humans. The term vitamin B_{12} is now used as a generic descriptor for all corrinoids containing copper with cobalamin activity. Cyanocobalamin, although synthetic, is taken as the most representative compound of the vitamin B_{12} group. The basic structure of vitamin B_{12} consists of four pyrrole rings joined into a larger planar ring containing six conjugated double bonds. One cobalt ion is organically complexed at the centre of this structure to six atoms. These consist of four nitrogen atoms (one from each of the pyrrole rings), a fifth nitrogen atom from a long 5,6-dimethylbenzimidazole side chain and one other variable link. The fifth nitrogen and the variable link occur at points directly above and below the flat corrinoid ring axis. The cobalt atom at the centre carries one positive charge. Cobalt itself was discovered to be essential as a trace element for certain animals in the 1930's. However elemental cobalt is not essential for humans. But cobalt is also part of vitamin B_{12}. This is the only form required by humans.

There are three natural forms of vitamin B_{12}, namely adenosylcobalamin, methylcobalamin and hydroxocobalamin. Cyanocobalamin is an artifact produced during isolation of the vitamin where the variable link has been replaced by a cyano (–CN) group. In the body this group must be replaced by one of the natural links before the vitamin becomes biologically active. In adenosylcobalamin, the link becomes a 5'-deoxy-5'-adenosyl group (or simply adenosyl for short). In methylcobalamin, the link is a simple methyl (–CH$_3$) group. And in hydroxocobalamin, the link is a hydroxyl (–OH) group. The cyanide ion may also be replaced by other ions such as nitrite, sulphate and chloride. All these synthetic derivatives are equally active. There are over 20 naturally occurring analogues and over 50 biosynthetic derivatives of vitamin B_{12} known. The relative biopotency of a number of the more important forms are given in Table 56.1 for comparison. Vitamin B_{12} is a very stable vitamin. Chemists have termed vitamin B_{12} the biological Grignard reagent, because of its direct carbon-to-metal link in some forms.

Biological Functions

• Around 2 - 3 mg of vitamin B_{12} may be stored in the human body. Most of this occurs in the form of adenosylcobalamin in the liver. High concentrations of the vitamin also occur in the kidneys. The supply of vitamin B_{12} in the body is sufficient to last from about 2 years to possibly 5 years in some cases. In the liver, a protein called transcobalamin I combines with the available vitamin B_{12} to provide a long-term storage depot. This is the only known case of a genuine biological storage form for a water-soluble vitamin.

- There are two major coenzyme forms of vitamin B_{12} namely, methylcobalamin and 5'-deoxyadenosylcobalamin, or adenosylcobalamin for short. Methylcobalamin is formed in the cytoplasm whereas adenosylcobalamin is formed in the mitochondria. These are members of the alkyl cobalamins and the cobamide cobalamins, respectively. Other forms of the above coenzymes may occur rarely and research is continuing into their significance, if any, to human nutrition. These coenzymes are widely distributed in bacteria. However, in the human they are involved in only three known reactions namely, the methylation of the amino acid homocysteine, the conversion of methylmalonyl-CoA to succinyl-CoA, and the reversible conversion of leucine to Ⓐ-leucine.

- Hydroxocobalamin is the main transport form of vitamin B_{12} but it does not act as a coenzyme itself. In combination with the plasma carrier protein, transcobalamin II, it may enter the cells and dissociate to form methylcobalamin in the cytoplasm. It may alternatively enter the mitochondria where it dissociates to form adenosylcobalamin.

- Methylcobalamin is involved in methylation reactions which also involve the participation of folate as methyl-THFA. The enzyme involved is called methyltransferase and it converts homocysteine to methionine by the addition of a methyl ($-CH_3$) group which comes from the folate cofactor. The reaction is complex and may be considered to proceed as follows: methylene-THFA is converted to methyl-THFA, then in the presence of methylcobalamin and the enzyme methyltransferase, the methyl group on the folate coenzyme is transferred to the sulfur atom of homocysteine to form methionine. Methionine can go on to form S-adenosylmethionine which is the ubiquitous methyl group donor in many important synthetic reactions in the body. However, in the absence of vitamin B_{12} there is a buildup of methyl-THFA which is known as the tetrahydrofolate trap, because it results in a relative deficiency of utilisable folic acid.

- Adenosylcobalamin is involved in molecular rearrangements which are catalysed by an enzyme called mutase. The isomerism of methylmalonic acid to succinic acid is an example. This reaction involves adenosylcobalamin together with the pantothenic acid cofactor, CoA.

- Lesser quantities of unusual derivatives of vitamin B_{12} may act as coenzymes in certain bacteria. These are sometimes termed pseudocobalamins, but they are probably of no significance in human metabolism.

- Through its metabolic reactions as outlined above, vitamin B_{12} is involved in areas of carbohydrate, lipid and amino acid metabolism, in the production of red blood cells, and in maintaining the integrity of the nervous system by ensuring the formation of the protective myelin sheath surrounding nerve axons.

- Vitamin B_{12} maintains glutathione in the reduced state. This tripeptide, consists of glutamic acid, cysteine and glycine moieties, and is involved in protecting various enzymes from oxidation in the body.

- Vitamin B_{12} may serve to detoxify traces of cyanide in food and inhaled tobacco smoke.

Requirement

The average intake of cobalt itself ranges from 5 to 8 µg per day. But free cobalt even in high concentrations cannot provide a substitute for vitamin B_{12} in the human. In other animals, such as ruminants, all their vitamin B_{12}, indeed all their B-group vitamin requirements, can usually be met because their rumen bacteria not only synthesise all these vitamins but also supply the needs of the animals in most cases. In humans, the average intake of vitamin B_{12} ranges from 5 to 15 µg per day, with extreme values from about 1 to 1,000 μg in some cases. A small percentage (less than 3 percent) is absorbed by simple diffusion. The rest requires the glycoprotein carrier, called intrinsic factor, which is secreted in the stomach. This mechanism may allow up to 10 μg per to be absorbed from the small intestine. On daily intakes, up to 3 μg, some 50 percent of the vitamin B_{12} in the diet is absorbed on average. In normal individuals, the daily turnover of vitamin B_{12} ranges from about 0.5 to 2.5 μg. There appears to be an obligatory loss of about one-thousandth of the total body stores of the vitamin per day.

The recommended adult daily intake of vitamin B_{12} in both males and in females is 2.4 μg/d. These intakes are sufficient to maintain normal serum levels of the vitamin in the majority of individuals. Some older people do not absorb vitamin B_{12} efficiently, so it is advisable for people over 50 years of age to ensure their Vitamin B_{12} intake with fortified foods or supplements.

Long-term studies on vitamin B_{12} are difficult to maintain as it may take up to five years for deficiency signs to emerge in some individuals. Judging from studies on the remission of pernicious anaemia, the minimum daily requirement of the vitamin is probably in the range 0.1 to 1.0 μg, with the upper value giving optimal responses. With very few exceptions, animal foods such as meat particularly liver and kidney, and milk are the best sources of vitamin B_{12}. The compendium gives further details in this regard (Table 56.2).

Toxicity

Vitamin B_{12} is probably one of the safest of all the vitamins. There is no known toxicity of vitamin B_{12} when taken orally. In a few cases, injections of the vitamin have caused allergic reactions. Excessive intake of vitamin B_{12} is unlikely to cause an imbalance of other B-group vitamins because of the much greater concentration of these vitamins in the body. Excess vitamin B_{12} is taken up by the liver and excreted in the bile.

Cobalt itself is toxic in high doses. When intake exceed 30 µg per day, toxic effects including goitre, insufficient thyroxine and ultimately death may occur. Intakes of about 20µg per day (as may occur with certain heavy beer drinkers!) may result in the over-production of red blood cells (polycythaemia) and possibly cardiovascular disease. High protein intakes may protect against some symptoms of cobalt intoxication.

Deficiency

A deficiency of vitamin B_{12} may take from 2 to years to 5 years to develop in humans. This is because the liver can store relatively large amounts of the vitamin, and its requirement amounts to only about 1 µg per day or less in most adults. Also, the blood level of vitamin B_{12} may fall to 20 percent of its normal level before clinical symptoms develop. These symptoms include anaemia and neurological disorders. The anaemia of vitamin B_{12} deficiency has been termed pernicious anaemia and is characterised by a chronically reduced number of larger the normal red blood cells.

Certain patients with pernicious anaemia have been found to contain antibodies to the intrinsic factor. This may lead to atrophy of the gastric mucosa resulting in a lack of both intrinsic factor and HCl secretion (achlorhydria). However, it is not the lack of HCl, but the lack of intrinsic factor which is the primary cause of vitamin B_{12} deficiency. The intrinsic factor is a glycoprotein, that is a protein linked to a carbohydrate moiety, and is essential for the absorption of vitamin B_{12}, although it is not itself absorbed in the process. Other conditions that interfere with vitamin B_{12} absorption are chronic sprue and some rare intestinal disorders. The main symptoms accompanying pernicious anaemia are lack of energy due to physical and mental feelings of fatigue. In the absence of vitamin B_{12}, methyl-THFA builds up in the body and thymine synthesis is impaired. The buildup of methyl-THFA is a trap which in effect causes a secondary deficiency of folate and it is this which ultimately results in macrocytic anaemia. This anaemia is the same as that resulting from a primary folate deficiency, but has been termed pernicious anaemia because oral administration of vitamin B_{12} often failed to correct the disorder in the past. Nowadays, supplements of vitamin B_{12} in the range 200 to 1,000 μg per day are frequently sufficient to offset the lack of intrinsic factor. Failing this, injections of the vitamin at regular intervals should prove beneficial. It has been suggested that calcium may assist in the absorption of vitamin B_{12}.

Doses of folic acid in excess of 500 μg per day may also correct the symptoms of pernicious anaemia but cannot halt the neurological changes associated with vitamin B_{12} deficiency. Initial symptoms of peripheral neuropathy include weakness in the arms and legs, poor reflexes and impaired sensory perception. The gait may become unsteady and stammering may develop. Soreness, stiffness, pins and needles, numbness and ultimately paralysis may occur. Severe psychotic symptoms, resembling schizophrenia may also develop. Mental symptoms such as poor memory and moodiness are often the first symptoms of vitamin B_{12} deficiency.

With time, some of the neurological damage caused by a lack of vitamin B_{12} may be irreversible, hence the urgency of administering vitamin B_{12} in cases of pernicious anaemia, even in doubtful cases. In some rare disorders where the formation of the adenosylcobalamin coenzyme is impaired, there may be a buildup of methylmalonic acid unless high doses of vitamin B_{12} are administered. Doses up to 1,000 times the normal daily intake are required to overcome this defect. In an even rarer defect of the transport protein, transcobalamin II, there may be a deficiency of both coenzyme forms and methylmalonate and homocysteine may both appear in the urine.

In some animals, a deficiency of vitamin B_{12} results in poor growth rates. In hens, a deficiency results in poor hatching of eggs. Interestingly, anaemia is rarely associated with vitamin B_{12} deficiency in animals.

Table 56.1. Relative biopotency of different forms of vitamin B_{12}

NAME	NOMINAL VALUE (percent)
Natural forms	
Adenosylcobalamin	100
Methylcobalamin	100
Hydroxocobalamin	100
Aquocobalamin	100
Synthetic forms	
Cyanocobalamin	100
Other derivatives such as: Nitrite, Sulphite, Sulphate, Chloride, etc.	100

Although there are differences in activity of different analogues depending on the route of administration or the laboratory test used to assay the activity, all forms are equally effective in the body itself. Cyanocobalamin is the most stable and widely used supplementary form. Adenosyl- and methyl- cobalamin are the natural coenzyme forms. Because of the relatively massive size of the vitamin B_{12} structure, all forms have approximately the same theoretical biopotencies. Hydroxo- and aquo- cobalamin are virtually identical forms that differ only by a single hydrogen atom; the aquo- form carries a full water molecule (H_2O) instead of a hydroxyl group (–OH). They are depot forms in the red blood cell and in the liver (and were previously termed vitamins B_{12a} and B_{12b}, respectively). Adenosylcobalamin is also a depot form found mainly in red blood cells, liver and kidney. In contrast, methylcobalamin is the main cobalamin found in the blood plasma.

Table 56.2. Vitamin B_{12} compendium

FOOD GROUP	VITAMIN B_{12} LEVEL
Milk and products	Very low
Eggs	Very low
Meat and fish	Very variable
Fats and oils	Nil
Grain and products	Nil, variable
Nuts and pulses	Nil, variable
Root vegetables	Nil, variable
Leaf vegetables	Nil
Fruit	Nil
Sweets	Nil

57

Vitamin E

Common Names

Vitamin E.
α–Tocopherol.

Alternative names

d-alpha-Tocopherol.
Tocopherols (alpha-, beta-, gamma-, delta-, epsilon-, zeta-1, zeta-2 and eta-; or α–, β–, γ–, δ–, ε–, ζ_1–, ζ_2– and η–).
ζ_1-or ζ_2-Tocopherol are the same and now called α-tocotrienol.
ε-Tocopherol is now called β-tocotrienol.
η-Tocopherol is now called γ-tocotrienol.
The fourth tocotrienol is called δ-tocotrienol.
Tocotrienols (alpha-, beta-, gamma-, delta-).
The E vitamins. E_1, E_2, E_3. The E group.
Anti-oxidant vitamin. Rat antisterility vitamin. Antisterility factor.
The fertility vitamin. The vitality vitamin.
Tocochromanol-3. Plastochromanol-3. Factor X.

Some of the above terms are obsolete or trivial.

History

1922: Evans and Bishop reported a 'Factor X' in wheat that prevented foetal resorption (sterility) in rats. Mattill finds the same factor in yeast and lettuce.

1923: Evans, *et al.*, find 'X' in various oils.

1924: Sure changes the designation to vitamin E (the next letter free at the time).

1925: This factor had also been purified by Emerson in 1925.

1936: The first pure extract of vitamin E was isolated by Evans, *et al.*, and shown to be a tocopherol. In the same year, several different tocopherols are isolated. The most active is designated α–tocopherol.

1938: The structure of α–tocopherol was established by Fernholtz. The vitamin was synthesised by Karrer.

1956: By 1956, seven tocopherols had been isolated and, in that year, Green found yet another. It is now known that four of these are tocopherols and the other four are tocotrienols.

-----: Vitamin E is now a generic term for all tocopherols and tocotrienols with the qualitative biological activity of α–tocopherol. The term tocopherol is specifically reserved for the tocol derivatives with vitamin E activity but does not include the tocotrienols. The measure tocopherol equivalent (mg TE) includes the contribution of all vitamin E derivatives (tocopherols and tocotrienols) with the qualitative biological activity of α–tocopherol. Vitamin E is a fat-soluble vitamin.

There are four members of the fat-soluble vitamins as listed in Fig. 57.1.

Fig. 57.1. The Fat-Soluble Vitamins

- Vitamin E
- Vitamin A
- Vitamin K
- Vitamin D

Each of these will be considered in detail in the following chapters.

Nature

There is some confusion in the text books over the correct chemical names of the various vitamin E compounds. This is in part due to the large number of chemical substitutions that can occur and partly because of the inaccurate classifications used in the past. To clear up this difficulty, it is worth adding a separate table, at the outset, giving the currently accepted common names and the corresponding chemical names of each of the eight naturally occurring compounds (Table 57.1). A wide range of other methyl- substituted forms of vitamin E may be formed by chemical reaction. These changes generally result in loss of activity and are of no interest in nutrition. Vitamin E is a relatively unstable vitamin.

Vitamin E is synthesised by plants and many microorganisms. There are eight naturally occurring compounds with vitamin activity. Four of these are tocopherols and four are tocotrienols. Chemically, they are all isoprenoid substituted 6-hydroxychromanes, or tocols for short, and all are lipid-soluble compounds. The most active of these is d-α-tocopherol (more specifically with the absolute configuration 2R,4'R,8'R-α-tocopherol, or RRR–α-tocopherol) which is seen as the most representative compound of the vitamin E group. The term vitamin E is now used as a generic descriptor for all tocopherols or tocotrienols with α–tocopherol activity.

The relative potencies of the natural forms of vitamin are illustrated in Table 57.2. These biopotency values are somewhat arbitrary and, like all such values, vary considerably depending on the specific test used to establish them. As a general rule, the antioxidant properties of these substances are inversely related to their biopotencies. Hence, δ-tocopherol is the most powerful antioxidant while being the least biologically active compound, whereas the opposite holds true for α–tocopherol.

Older units give vitamin activity in terms of international units (IU), which were based on biological activity tests. However, because of improvements in the direct chemical measurement of vitamin E compounds, these older units can now be replaced by α–tocopherol equivalents (or simply tocopherol equivalents), where by definition 1 α–tocopherol equivalent, or mg TE, equals 1.49 international units of vitamin E activity exactly.

More conveniently, the practical relationship is used:

$$3 \text{ IU} = 2 \text{ mg TE} = 2 \text{ mg } \alpha\text{-tocopherol}$$

By definition, one tocopherol equivalent (TE) corresponds to the activity of one milligram of α-tocopherol. Following the above definition, it is possible to assign fractional tocopherol equivalents to less potent forms of vitamin E. Taking α-tocopherol as having 1.0 TE per mg; β-tocopherol is said to have 0.5, γ-tocopherol is said to have 0.1, and α-tocotrienol is said to have 0.3 TE per mg, respectively. Other values for the naturally occurring forms of vitamin E are also given in Table 57.2. Many isomers and esters of vitamin E, used mainly as supplements, are also active and some of the most common are listed in Table 57.3.

Biological Functions

- Vitamin E acts as a potent lipid-soluble antioxidant. This property seems to be inversely related to the biological potency of different forms of vitamin E. Vitamin E helps to prevent the peroxidation of cell membranes. Together with the selenium-dependent enzyme, glutathione peroxidase, it minimises cellular and subcellular damage. This is important not only for the cell membrane itself but also for membranes surrounding various organelles. Vitamin E is concentrated in cell membranes, particularly in mitochondrial membranes. Other enzymes that play a role in protecting the cell against oxidising agents include glutathione reductase, superoxide dismutase and catalase. Glutathione itself is an important tripeptide which contains the sulphur containing amino acid cysteine.

- Selenium reduces the requirement for vitamin E in a number of ways. It helps to promote the efficient absorption of vitamin E in the diet by maintaining the production of pancreatic juice and hence the absorption of fat. It helps to conserve blood levels of vitamin E through an unknown mechanism. And it cooperates with vitamin E in protecting cell membranes by promoting the action of certain enzymes. By the same token, a high level of vitamin E reduces the overall requirement for selenium. Interestingly, vitamin C also has some selenium sparing action.

- It is believed that vitamin E plays a role in certain aspects of cell membrane metabolism other than merely acting as an antioxidant, but this role remains to be elucidated. Indeed, this may prove to be the key to the real essential function of vitamin E in the body.

- Vitamin E, in its capacity as an antioxidant, also protects certain essential nutrients from breaking down. These include vitamin C, vitamin A, and various amino acids and polyunsaturated fatty acids. Vitamin E and vitamin C may act to reinforce each other's antioxidant ability.

- Vitamin E may help to maintain the integrity of various nucleic acids and thereby reduce their turnover rates. On the other hand, the effect may be indirectly related to the decrease in red blood cell survival time which prompts the release of the blood forming hormone erythropoietin from the kidney, thus increasing synthesis in certain bone marrow cells during vitamin E deficiency. Vitamin E also influences the level of the purine-metabolising enzyme xanthine oxidase. And this action involves not only DNA and RNA but also protein synthesis.

- Vitamin E reduces the overall oxygen uptake by various tissues including muscle and nerve by preventing peroxidation. Vitamin E also influences the level of the muscle enzyme creatine kinase and, therefore, is required for the normal development and maintenance of muscle tissue.

- The primary oxidation product of vitamin E is the tocopheroxyl radical. Although certain forms of vitamin E are reversibly oxidised and reduced, they do not normally participate in electron transport systems. On the other hand, the electron transport chain can reduce tocopheroxyl radicals, so it may have an important physiological role in recycling vitamin E.

- Vitamin E may improve the circulation in certain individuals. This may be of benefit to certain arthritic patients who suffer from recurrent leg cramps (intermittent claudication).

- Vitamin E, together with several other antioxidant nutrients, may help to prevent coronary heart disease. In particular, it is beneficial in certain cases of angina.

- It has been claimed that vitamin E may improve the healing of wounds and burns and minimise the formation of scar tissue.

- High doses of vitamin E appear to have an anti-ageing effect in certain laboratory animals by promoting longevity. Vitamin E has been termed the vitality vitamin because of speculative claims that it can make one look younger. This is not true. What is certain, however, is that the vitamin may delay some damaging (ageing) effects produced by free radicles originating from radiation or pollution. Vitamin E also protects the lungs from the effects of air pollution.

- Because of its role in preserving polyunsaturated fatty acids, vitamin E, has a role to play in maintaining the essential fatty acid level in the body and, therefore, in ensuring adequate substrates for prostaglandin formation. On the other hand, because it acts as an antioxidant it may inhibit the formation of some prostaglandin-like substances while enhancing the formation of others.

- Vitamin E can act as an anticoagulant and may increase the risk of bleeding problems. For example, there is some evidence that vitamin E inhibits blood platelet aggregation, possibly by inhibiting thromboxane formation.

- Because of its relatively high concentration in the pituitary gland, the adrenal glands and in the testes, it has been suggested that vitamin E may protect certain hormones produced in these glands, but this theory is not proven.

- Vitamin E is required for fertility in several animals but not in the human. The cow, the hen and the rat are among those animals which depend on vitamin E for this function.

- Vitamin E may have a role to play in promoting antibody

formation and in maintaining the vigour of certain white blood cells, and hence the immune system.

• Vitamin E may have a non-antioxidant function as a cell signaling molecule. α–Tocopherol modulates two major signal transduction pathways centered on protein kinase C and phosphatidylinositol 3-kinase.

• Vitamin E may also act as a regulator of gene expression.

• Vitamin E appears to slow down the rate of development of certain types of experimental cancer cells.

Requirement

Good sources of vitamin E include margarine, butter, eggs, wheat germ and vegetables. Liver and oily fish are also excellent sources. Vegetable oils are by far the best sources of vitamin E. The requirement for vitamin E is related to the amount of polyunsaturated fatty acids in the diet, or more generally the ratio of oxidants to antioxidants in the body. Excessive intake of oxidants will necessitate a corresponding increase in the vitamin E intake. Selenium and vitamin C exert a sparing action on vitamin E. Bile promotes the absorption of lipids and hence vitamin E. Under normal conditions it appears that an average intake of some 4 to 9 mg of α–tocopherol (or 4 to 9 tocopherol equivalents of vitamin E activity) is adequate. Additional vitamin E may be required in certain circumstances, such as in elderly persons suffering from circulatory disturbances. But virtually all adult diets supply sufficient vitamin E. The recommended adult daily intake of vitamin E in both males and in females is 15 mg/d.

α–Tocopherol is the major contributor to vitamin E activity in both plant and animal foods. In plants, significant contributions to the total activity are made most often by γ–tocopherol, although all forms are known to occur. The content of vitamin E varies widely in foodstuffs. The analysis of different forms of vitamin E in food is ongoing. However, the compendium gives a general picture (Table 57.4).

Vitamin E is absorbed from the small intestine and is transported together with lipid to the liver. It is distributed to various tissues by associating with lipoproteins in the blood. Vitamin E is stored mainly unchanged in various tissues but particularly in adipose tissue. The main route of excretion of vitamin E is in the faeces.

Toxicity

Vitamin E is essentially non-toxic. In a number of persons who consumed up to 500 mg α–tocopherol per day for 3 years, no symptoms were evident. Supplements of vitamin E up to 700 mg per day only produced minor symptoms in about 1 percent of individuals. Minor symptoms of toxicity may include diarrhoea, dermatitis, fatigue, and palpitations. Very occasionally a transient increase in blood pressure has been observed with high doses. Continuous use of over 1,500 mg per day is inadvisable. High doses of vitamin E tend to worsen the symptoms of vitamin K deficiency in humans but have no effect on blood clotting in normal individuals.

Sudden increases (or decreases) of vitamin E intake are inadvisable. High intakes should be avoided by patients with certain illnesses, particularly those with rheumatic heart disease, high blood pressure, diabetes or hyperactive thyroid function. Supplements of vitamin E are often labelled in international units (IU). The ideal way to take supplements of vitamin is to increase the intake starting from 100 or 200 IU and buildup gradually in steps of 100 or 200 IU up to a maximum of 600 to 1,000 IU for men, or about 400 to 600 IU for women. Likewise, when finishing a course one should step down the dose gradually. It should be pointed out, however, that unless vitamin E is recommended for a specific condition it is probably unnecessary to take any supplements.

Deficiency

Vitamin E has been termed the vitamin in search of a disease. Although sterility is a dramatic effect of vitamin E deficiency in certain animals, notably the rat, no such effect is evident in the human. However, recent research has shown that vitamin E deficiency in humans can be induced experimentally by feeding vitamin-free diets high in polyunsaturated fatty acids and low in selenium. Like all other lipid-soluble vitamins, vitamin E deficiency may also arise as a result of impaired fat absorption. Apart from this, vitamin E deficiency is extremely rare in humans, except for some infants who occasionally suffer from a deficiency.

The main symptoms of vitamin E deficiency are increased fragility of the red blood cells and muscular weakness which is sometimes accompanied by the appearance of creatinine in the urine. Creatinine is a breakdown product of muscle activity but is normally present only in small amounts. Vitamin E deficiency results in increased peroxidation of cell membrane lipids resulting in abnormalities in membrane transport and a decrease in mitochondrial energy production. In vitamin E-deficient cells, an increased mutation rate due to oxidation of DNA is also commonly observed. In general, there is a reduced ability to cope with various forms of pollution, stress and disease. Oxidised fats occasionally appear which are pigmented and occur in older animals as well as during vitamin E deficiencies. In certain animals, deficiency of vitamin E leads to a form of muscular dystrophy. This condition however is not the same as human muscular dystrophy. Vitamin E therapy has occasionally been used to ease muscle pain, including the pain of angina and even premenstrual tension. A vitamin E deficiency is common in premature babies and haemolytic anaemia may occur, as a result, unless vitamin E is administered. This is perhaps the clearest case of a disease produced by vitamin E deficiency in humans. Anaemia is not associated with adult deficiencies, even though the red blood cell life span is slightly reduced. An increased fragility of red blood cells in adults has also been noted. This may result in a tendency to cause haemolysis more easily in the presence of peroxides.

In some cases of lipoprotein disorders, vitamin E deficiency may occur, presumably because under normal conditions vitamin E is transported mainly in combination with the lipoproteins and, in particular, the $\alpha-$ and $\beta-$ lipoprotein fraction in the blood. In many cases of vitamin E deficiency, the mitochondrion is one of the first cell organelles to be damaged. The levels of vitamin E in various tissues is lower than normal in patients with cystic fibrosis. The significance of this finding is under detailed investigation at the present time.

In one study, human volunteers who were maintained on a dietary level of only 2 to 3 tocopherol equivalents of vitamin E per day for up to 2 years did not develop a frank deficiency disease, although their blood levels of the vitamin were reduced by over 50 percent and their red blood cells were more fragile than normal. These effects would have developed somewhat faster on a completely vitamin E-free diet. The most accurate indication of vitamin E deficiency in humans is not the presence of disease or even the level of the vitamin in the blood *per se*, but the ratio of the vitamin to the total plasma lipid. This value should not be lower than 0.8 mg □-tocopherol per gram of plasma lipid.

In the vitamin E-deficient female rat, ovulation and fertilisation are normal, but at a later stage in the pregnancy, the foetus fails. In the male rat sterility results, initially because of a decreased sperm motility, and later because of damage to the testes. Despite the widespread myth that vitamin E is also a human fertility factor, if not a downright aphrodisiac, there is absolutely no evidence for this belief other than perhaps in the minds of certain vitamin E purveyors. In some animals, including the rat, prolonged deficiency of vitamin also results in kidney damage. Liver damage may also occur but this is prevented by administering selenium or sulphur containing amino acids such as cysteine or methionine. Indirectly, a vitamin A deficiency may occur as a consequence of a vitamin E deficiency. This is because the antioxidant property of vitamin E normally protects vitamin A from oxidation in the body.

Table 57.1. Composition of different forms of vitamin E

COMMON NAME	CHEMICAL NAME
Saturated forms	
α–Tocopherol	5,7,8-Trimethyltocopherol
β–Tocopherol	5,8-Dimethyltocopherol
γ–Tocopherol	7,8-Dimethyltocopherol
δ–Tocopherol	8-Methyltocopherol
Unsaturated forms	
α–Tocotrienol	5,7,8-Trimethyltocotrienol
β–Tocotrienol	5,8-Dimethyltocotrienol
γ–Tocotrienol	7,8-Dimethyltocotrienol
δ–Tocotrienol	8-Methyltocotrienol

There are eight different isoforms of vitamin E that belong to two categories, four saturated analogues called tocopherols (α, β, γ, and δ) and four unsaturated analogues called tocotrienols (α, β, γ, and δ). All of these consist of the dextrorotatory, d-, enantiomers only.

Table 57.2. Relative biopotency of different natural forms
of vitamin E

NAME	TOCOPHEROL EQUIVALENT (µg giving one µg TE)	NOMINAL VALUE (percent)
α–Tocopherol	1	100
β–Tocopherol	2	50
γ–Tocopherol	10	10
δ–Tocopherol	100	1
α–Tocotrienol	3.3	30
β–Tocotrienol	20	5
γ–Tocotrienol	-----	Negligible
δ–Tocotrienol	-----	Negligible
Unspecified mixture (not including α–Tocopherol)	5	20

A large range of substances with some similarities to the tocopherols also exhibit vitamin E activity. These include ubiquinone derivatives; quinones, phenols, chromanes and coumarins. It is interesting to note that a derivative of ubiquinone (CoQ_{10}) and ubichromenol have at least 100 percent activity on the above scale. Another substance, N,N'-diphenyl-p-phenylenediamine, can prevent signs of vitamin E deficiency in certain experimental animals. Methylene blue and thiodiphenyamine also prevent such symptoms. All these substances inhibit the oxidation of polyunsaturated fatty acids but cannot completely substitute for vitamin E. Any major change in the chemical structure of vitamin E results in a loss of biological activity.

Table 57.3. Relative biopotency of different isomers and esters
of α–tocopherol

NAME	OLD SCALE [1] (IU per mg)	NOMINAL VALUE (percent)
d-α-Tocopherol	1.49	100
d-α-Tocopheryl acetate	1.36	90
d-α-Tocopheryl succinate	1.21	80
dl-rac-α-Tocopherol	1.10	74
dl-rac-α-Tocopheryl acetate [2]	1.00	67
dl-rac-α-Tocopheryl succinate	0.89	60

1. The IU scale is converted to the TE scale by multiplying by 0.67.

2. An older semi-synthetic form, consisting of 50% d-α–tocopherol acetate and 50% other isomers called 2-ambo-α–tocopheryl acetate, is no longer available. The modern synthetic form consists of an equal mixture of all eight isomers—a racemic mixture with equal amounts of d- and l- optical isomers called *all-rac-*α–tocopherol (commonly labelled as dl-*rac*-α–tocopherol).

Table 57.4. Vitamin E compendium

FOOD GROUP	VITAMIN E LEVEL
Milk and products	Very low
Eggs	Medium
Meat and fish	Medium, variable
Fats and oils	Very high, variable
Grain and products	Medium, variable
Nuts / Pulses	Very high / Low
Root vegetables	Low, variable
Leaf vegetables	Low
Fruit	Very low
Sweets	Nil

58

Vitamin A (and the Carotenoids)

Common names

Vitamin A.
Retinol.

Alternative names

The A vitamins (or group).
Preformed vitamin A.
Vitamin A_1 (all-*trans*). A_1 alcohol.
Retinal. Retinine$_1$.
Vitamin A_2. Retinol$_2$.
3-dehydroretinol. 3-dehydroretinal.
Retinoic acid.
Antixerophthalmic factor. Lard factor. Biosterol. Oleovitamin A.
Axerophthol. Anti-infective vitamin. Epithelial protection vitamin.
Neovitamin A. Neo-β-vitamin A_1.
(Also various derivatives, such as esters.)
Provitamin A. Vitamin A precursor.
Carotene. Beta-carotene (β–Carotene). Carotenoids.

Many of the above designations are obsolete.

History

circa 1500 BC: The Ancient Egyptians cured night blindness using liver juice.

circa 430 BC: Hippocrates records this same effect.

1831: Wachen proposed the term "carotene" for a pigment crystallized from carrot roots.

1837: Berzelius gave the name '*xanthophylls*' (originally phylloxanthins) to yellow polar pigments extracted from autumn leaves.

1842: Budd explained how dry eyes could be cured with animal food.

1907: Willstatter established the empirical formula of carotenoids (C40).

1911: Tswett separated many pigments using chromatography and called them 'carotenoids'.

1912: Hopkins suggested that a factor in milk was required for growth in rats.

1913: Osborne and Mendel demonstrate that the milk factor is fat-soluble and present in several fats.

1915: McCollum and Davis coin the term 'fat-soluble A' (as distinct from 'water-soluble B', which cured Beriberi). By this time Osborn and Mendel had shown that cod-liver oil contains the factor.

1917: McCollum and Simmonds show that xerophthalmia in rats is due to the lack of 'fat-soluble A'.

1919: Steenbook discovers carotene possesses antixerophthalmia activity in rats.

1920: Drummond coins the term Vitamin A

circa 1930: Moore shows that carotene is a precursor of Vitamin A. Karrer, *et al.*, discover the structure of β-carotene.

1935: Wald discovers that the visual pigment, rhodopsin, in the retina of the eye contains Vitamin A, hence the name retinol.

1937: By this time, Holmes and Corbett have isolated and crystallised pure Vitamin A. Karrer *et al.*, have also synthesised Vitamin A.

-----: It is now known that there are several forms of Vitamin A. The term Vitamin A is now used as a generic descriptor for all β-ionone derivatives (except provitamin A carotenoids) with the qualitative biological activity of retinol. Vitamin A activity is measured in retinol activity equivalents (RAE) which may include the contribution of β-carotene and other provitamins to the total activity.

The term retinoids includes both the natural and synthetic forms of Vitamin A.

Nature

Vitamin A is a derivative of certain plant carotenoids. These provitamins can be converted to vitamin A in the human body. Carotenoids consist of a group of pigments containing 40 carbon atoms and are identical in their middle structure of 18 carbon atoms. They consist of a continuous system of conjugated double bonds called a polyene chain sequence, and can be considered chemically as being built up of isoprene units. Vitamin A and the carotenoids themselves are all lipid-soluble compounds. The carotenoids only occur in plants, where they are synthesised. Vitamin A, however, only occurs in animal tissues, where it derives from the provitamin A carotenoids, and where it may be esterified and stored.

Retinol is taken as the most representative compound of the vitamin A group. Retinol itself is chemically a polyisoprenoid compound containing a cyclohexenyl (β–ionone) ring. In all, it consists of 20 carbon atoms, which is just half the number in β-carotene. It has a side chain consisting of 11 carbon atoms which is unsaturated and methylated. The double bonds of the side chain may exist in two conformations called *cis* or *trans*. As a rule, the *trans* forms are more active biologically than the *cis* forms, and the conformation of the central double bond is the most important. Tables 58.1 to 58.3 give the biopotencies of some *cis* and *trans* forms of vitamin A and a number of carotenoids, respectively.

It should be noted that there has been a change in the numbering system for atoms in the vitamin A side chain. In the past, the side chain carbon atoms were numbered from 7 to 15 away from the ring. Now these atom positions are numbered from 1' to 9', respectively. (The numbering of atoms in the ring has also been changed). Consequently, a derivative, found in the retina for example, which was previously termed 11-*cis*-retinal is now called 3'-*cis*-retinal, and so on. Many other derivatives of vitamin A are found in nature, such as 5,6-epoxyretinol, anhydroretinol and 4-ketoretinol, which have some biological activity but are not nutritionally dominant forms.

Retinol is occasionally termed vitamin A_1, to distinguish it from 3-dehydroretinol which is termed vitamin A_2, but these terms are falling into disuse. Alternatively, the terms $retinol_1$ and $retinol_2$ have been used to distinguish them. Retinol has previously been termed axerophthol. Retinal has also been termed retinene. Retinol, retinal and retinoic acid have also been termed vitamin A_1 alcohol, aldehyde and acid, respectively.

Over 700 carotenoids have been found to occur in nature but only about 50 of these have biological activity. Just as in the case of vitamin A itself, esters of the carotenoids have proportionately lower biological activity per unit mass than the free carotenoid forms. It is not relevant to indicate these values here. A large number of carotenoids such as xanthophyll, lycopene and zeaxanthin do not contribute to vitamin A activity because they do not contain a β–ionone ring structure.

The conversion of various carotenes to vitamin A in the body is limited. For example, the conversion of β–carotene in humans which gives rise to two molecules of retinol per molecule of β–carotene is at most only about 50 percent efficient. Furthermore, intestinal absorption is very variable and, on average, only a small percent of the provitamin A ingested is absorbed. Therefore, only a fraction of the β–carotene can be utilised to form retinol. Other provitamin A carotenoids yield even less retinol per molecule. In general, they are only about half as active again when compared with β–carotene. Vitamin A, including the carotenoids, are relatively stable compounds.

The most recent international standard measure for vitamin A activity, adopted in 2001, is the retinol activity equivalent (RAE). The retinol activity equivalent is a measure of vitamin A activity based on the capacity of the body to convert provitamin A carotenoids to retinal. These carotenoids must contain at least one unsubstituted ionone ring. Retinol can be easily oxidised to retinal or reduced to retinoic acid. all-*trans*-Retinol is now taken as the standard reference compound, and one microgram of retinol activity equivalent is defined as the activity of exactly one microgram of this form of vitamin A.

Preformed vitamin A is effectively absorbed and stored in the form of retinol, but provitamin A carotenoids are less easily digested and absorbed, and must be converted to retinol and other retinoids by the body after uptake. However, the efficiency of conversion of provitamin A carotenoids into retinol is highly variable, depending on the dietary source and its preparation, and on the overall digestive and absorptive capacities. Newer research has shown that the absorption of provitamin A carotenoids is only half as much as was previously believed. So, fruit and vegetables are not as useful for obtaining vitamin A as was previously believed.

As given in Table 58.4, the following relationships now hold:

$$
\begin{aligned}
1\ \mu g\ RAE \quad &=\quad 1\ \mu g\ retinol \\
&=\quad 2\ \mu g\ \beta\text{-carotene in oil} \\
&=\quad 12\ \mu g\ \beta\text{-carotene in food} \\
&=\quad 24\ \mu g\ other\ provitamin\ A\ carotenoids
\end{aligned}
$$

Although, in practice, there are variations in these ratios, in order to standardise the conversions, they are now accepted by definition. The relative biopotencies of various forms of vitamin A and the carotenoids in the human are listed in Table 58.5. The corresponding biopotencies in different animals are given in Table 58.6.

The term retinoids is occasionally used as a generic descriptor for all substances, both natural and synthetic, that exhibit retinol activity. The term vitamin A is mainly used as a generic descriptor for all natural β–ionone derivatives with retinol activity. The term deliberately excludes provitamin A carotenoids. However, the overall activity in the body includes the contribution of the provitamins.

Because there are several active metabolites of vitamin A, each with a specific range of functions, it is necessary to have some knowledge of the metabolism of the vitamin for a proper understanding of its varied functions. The overall picture of vitamin A metabolism is summarised in Figure 58.1, as follows:

Figure 58.1. Metabolic pathways arising from the metabolism of vitamin A and the carotenoids.

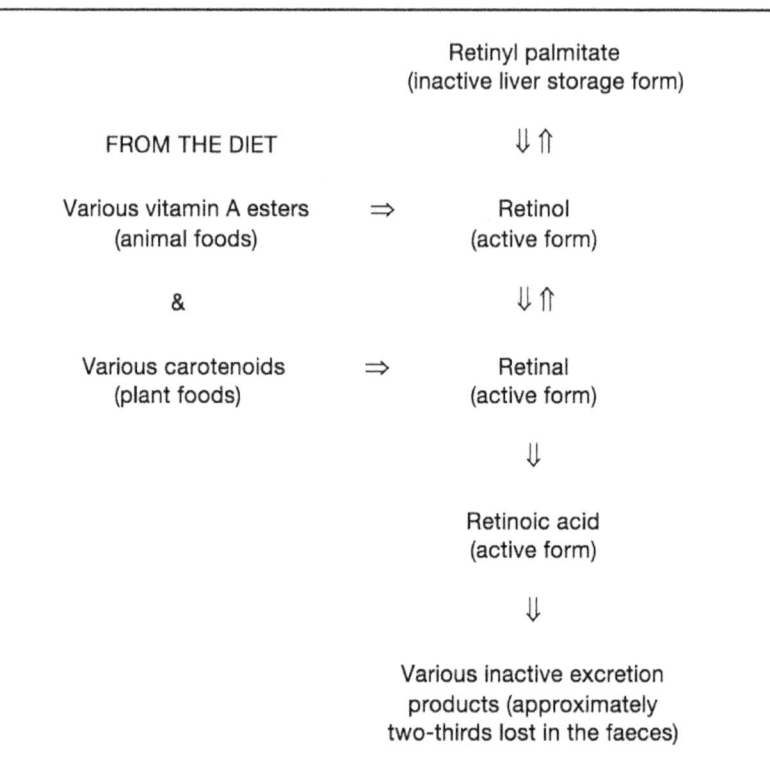

Retinyl palmitate
(inactive liver storage form)

FROM THE DIET   ⇓ ⇑

Various vitamin A esters   ⇒   Retinol
(animal foods)   (active form)

&   ⇓ ⇑

Various carotenoids   ⇒   Retinal
(plant foods)   (active form)

⇓

Retinoic acid
(active form)

⇓

Various inactive excretion
products (approximately
two-thirds lost in the faeces)

Biological Functions

- From the chemical point of view, retinol has the lowest oxidation state, retinal is next and retinoic acid has the highest oxidation state. These three main active forms of vitamin A have different functions in the body. In various target cells retinol is reversibly metabolised to retinal by the enzyme alcohol dehydrogenase. On the other hand, retinal is irreversibly metabolised to retinoic acid by various enzymes such as aldehyde oxygenase.

- In the human, the liver stores up to 95 percent of the vitamin A reserves mainly as palmitic acid ester. The esters are stored in fat droplets of specialised liver cells called hepatocytes. Liver may also contain traces of β–carotene although most of the β–carotene is stored in adipose tissue. In the hepatocyte, retinyl palmitate may be hydrolysed and mobilised by combining with a special carrier protein called apo-retinol-binding protein. After combining, the retinol/apo-retinol-binding protein complex is called holo-retinol-binding protein. The complex may leave the liver and circulate in the blood to bring the retinol to various tissues in the body.

- The apo-retinol-binding protein may also carry retinal, but only trace amounts of retinoic acid can associate with it. Another blood protein called prealbumin has a powerful affinity for the retinol carrying protein when retinol is present. It complexes with it to form a larger circulating complex that also carries the thyroid hormone thyroxine. For this reason, prealbumin has also been termed transthyretin.

- The holo-retinol-binding protein is recognised by cell surface receptors on various target tissues such as the intestine and the skin. It is believed that receptors are also present in other tissues such as the adrenal gland, the salivary gland and the testes. After attaching to the cell surface the bonding protein releases the retinol which enters the cell. There, once again, the retinol becomes attached to another specific protein called cellular retinol-binding protein (CRBP for short). It is believed that this intracellular protein protects vitamin A from oxidation and assists in its utilisation by the cell. Such cellular proteins are found in intestine, testes, liver, kidney, lung, brain and eye tissues. But they are not present in skeletal muscle or in the heart. Similarly, intracellular retinoic acid combines with a different protein called cellular retinoic acid-binding protein (CRABP for short). The amount of this protein in various cells depends on a number of factors including the age of the individual. The tissue distribution patterns of the retinol, and the retinoic acid-binding proteins are different and are not fully understood at the present time. No doubt, as a result of further research in this area, new facts about vitamin A will eventually emerge.

- In many ways retinol acts like a hormone. The simplest definition of a hormone is a substance that is produced in one part of the body, is secreted, and then travels in the blood stream to another part of the body called the target organ where it exerts its biological effect. The classical hormones regulate growth, metabolism and reproduction. They are produced in various endocrine glands in the body and secreted directly into the blood stream for transport to various sites. In recent years, a number of modifications of this concept have taken place to include such substances as local hormones and the like. It is not necessary to consider this definition further here but only to note that retinol and also some forms of vitamin D may now be considered as hormones in the general sense. Intracellular retinol in target cells may be transported to receptor sites on nuclear proteins. It is believed that some of its actions in stimulating growth may take place in a similar manner to those known for the steroid hormones. Retinal itself or retinoic acid do not appear to be capable of acting in this way. It has also been shown that vitamin A promotes the synthesis of RNA in certain cells in the gut and research on a vitamin A-dependent gene is well under way.

- Retinal is the main precursor of the visual pigments. The retina of the eye consists of rods and cones which are specialised cells connected to the optic nerve. The rods are specialised for vision in dim light and do not distinguish colour (rough vision), whereas the cones are adapted for bright light and colours (fine vision). It is believed that each cone contains one of three specific pigments sensitive to different wavelengths of light and hence contributes to the perception of a particular colour. Colour blindness may result from a defect in one or more of these pigments, each of which consists of a protein component and a retinal moiety. Three pigments are necessary to give full colour vision and these have been termed erythrolabe (red-sensitive), chlorolabe (green-sensitive) and cyanolabe (blue-sensitive), respectively. The theory of colour vision and the nature of colour blindness however, is outside the scope of a nutritional text.

- The rods contain a similar pigment called rhodopsin (or visual purple) which is several hundred times more sensitive to light and it is this pigment which allows dark adaptation to occur. When fully adapted, which takes about half an hour after going into darkness, the visual sensitivity to light may be increased by a factor of some 10,000 times. Rhodopsin also consists of a protein component called opsin and a retinal moiety. Rhodopsin is only operative in dim light when the retinal moiety is in the 3'-cis conformation. When light strikes rhodopsin the pigment is bleached and the 3'-cis-retinal is converted into the all-trans-retinal which then dissociates from the opsin. Subsequently, the 3'-cis-retinal form is regenerated and recombines with opsin to continue the process. An enzyme called retinal isomerase is required for this reaction but is not one-hundred percent efficient. Therefore, in the absence of sufficient additional vitamin A to maintain the requirement, night blindness may result. The conversion of all-trans-retinal to 3'-cis-retinal occurs in the eye. But some all-trans-retinal may be reduced to all-trans-retinol and travel to the liver. In the liver, this may be converted to 3'-cis-retinol and this in turn to 3'-cis-retinal, thus providing the required additional source of the active isomer which travels back to the eye. The above sequence of events has been termed the rhodopsin-vitamin A cycle.

- Retinol and retinal may be reversibly interconverted by the enzyme alcohol dehydrogenase. Therefore, either form may carry out the other's functions in the body.

- Retinoic acid, on the other hand, cannot be converted back to retinal or retinol in the body, hence cannot act as a substitute for them. However, retinoic acid itself has some very specific and unique functions. For example, when esterified to phosphoric acid, it is involved in the synthesis of glycoproteins (previously termed mucopolysaccharides). An interesting hypothesis has been put forward to explain its role in this process. It has been suggested that oligosaccharides (several mono-saccharides linked together) are transported across cell membranes by attaching to the trans form of esterified retinoic acid in the membrane. The complex then undergoes isomerisation to the cis form, thus enabling the oligosaccharide to cross the membrane. Chemically, the mechanism is similar to the isomerisation of all-*trans*- to *cis*- retinal in the vitamin A cycle.

- Retinoic acid cannot maintain night vision because it is not converted back to retinal in the body. But it has a number of other functions which are under investigation at present. These include growth and cell differentiation, the suppression of certain types of cancer cells and viruses, and the binding of mannose to liver glycoproteins. It has also been suggested that retinoic acid may be involved in the synthesis of certain steroid hormones in the adrenal cortex

- Through its various forms and functions, vitamin A is of great importance in the maintenance of normal health, growth, tissue repair, vision and reproduction. It promotes the efficient secretion of mucous fluid from certain cells in the mouth, respiratory tract, intestinal tract, urinary tract, female genital tract, prostate, seminal vesicles, eyes and paraocular glands. Through some of these functions, it is essential for reproduction, it promotes digestion, and it also acts to reduce the risk of infections and damage to the lungs from air pollutants. In general, vitamin A ensures the proper growth of bones and teeth. And it also promotes the growth of non-secretory cells such as those in the skin. In the latter regard, it has an important role in the keratinisation process.

- Specifically, vitamin A tends to stabilise various cellular membranes and, in particular, those of the intracellular organelles called lysosomes. It may also be involved in the release of proteolytic enzymes from these structures in the cell.

- Vitamin A is believed to be involved in maintaining the sense of smell and hence taste.

- Vitamin A may alleviate some of the symptoms of chronic alcohol abuse.

- Vitamin A may protect against certain forms of cancer and infections. It may also have a role to play in the immune response and in maintaining a healthy blood picture.

- Vitamin A has a rare role in transferring hydrogen ions (protons) across the cell membrane in certain purple bacteria. Such a process does not occur in animals however.

- β–Carotene itself has certain antioxidant properties.

- Three other carotenoids are important in maintaining the proper function of the macula in the eye. Lutein, zeaxanthin and *meso*-zeaxanthin are found in high concentrations in the human eye and protect the macula from degeneration. Apart from their antioxidant properties, they block blue light from reaching the underlying structures in the retina, thereby reducing the risk of light-induced oxidative damage that could lead to macular degeneration.

Requirement

The total vitamin A requirement may be provided in a typical Western diet as follows: some 37 percent of comes from meat, another 30 percent comes from vegetables (including vegetable oils) while about 14 percent is provided by milk and its products and another 14 percent comes from fruit. The vitamin A and carotenoid content of food varies widely and is subject to considerable losses during cooking and processing. Preformed vitamin A is derived from animal foods whereas carotenes are derived from plant foods. Anything from 10 up to 40 percent of the day-to-day vitamin A requirement may be provided as preformed vitamin A in the diet; an average value of around 30 percent is fairly typical. In many Western diets, therefore, about 70 percent of the vitamin A requirement is provided by the carotenoids. The ratio of vitamin A to carotenoid intake varies considerably from country to country and from season to season. Also, in some individual cases, for example vegetarians, practically all of the requirement must be obtained from the carotenoids.

The actual retinol equivalent of the carotenoids can vary depending on such factors as the bioavailability of the carotenoids, the amount of lipid in the food, and also the presence of other constituents in the diet. Vitamin A and the carotenoids may occur as esters in combination with phosphate, β-glucuronide, acetate, palmitate, or other long-chain fatty acids. Bile salts help break down these esters through a detergent action, and thus promote their absorption. Bile itself also promotes the absorption of fat and hence all fat-soluble vitamins. In animal sources, retinol is the chief esterified form, whereas in plant sources, β-carotene is the most significant nutritional form. A portion of the carotenes are broken down in the presence of bile salts and lecithin to yield retinal. In the gut mucosa, retinal is converted to retinol by the action of a reducing enzyme. The retinol combines with various long-chain fatty acids and is absorbed *via* the lymph. Gradually, the new esters enter the blood but are again removed by the liver and broken down. In the liver, the retinol is combined mainly with palmitate and stored in this form until required. Some retinal is oxidised to retinoic acid. Interestingly, the retinoic acid is absorbed directly into the blood stream but is not stored in the liver.

The vitamin A compendium (Table 58.7) summarizes the overall distribution of vitamin A (both actual and potential) in various foodstuffs. The recommended intakes are given in retinol activity equivalents (RAE), where 1 RAE is equivalent to 1 μg retinol. The values quoted include the possible contribution from β–carotene and other provitamin A carotenoids in the diet. See Table 58.4 for further details. The recommended adult daily intake of vitamin A in males is 900 μg RAE/d and in females is 700 μg RAE/d, respectively.

The vitamin A requirement is influenced by protein intake. There are two reasons for this. First, proteins reduce the surface tension of liquids and this physical effect, in itself, aids emulsification and absorption of fat droplets containing the vitamin. Second, a high protein diet stimulates the formation of an enzyme called β–carotene oxygenase in the mucosa. This enzyme splits the β–carotene to release active vitamin A. Interestingly, lipid itself also indirectly spares dietary vitamin A because it contains another fat-soluble vitamin, namely vitamin E, which acts as an antioxidant.

Various inactive metabolites of vitamin A are excreted in the faeces and in the urine. On average about 20 percent of the ingested vitamin

A is lost in the faeces within 2 days. The remaining 80 percent is absorbed and depending on a number of factors some 30 to 60 percent is stored in the liver. The 10 to 20 percent which is not stored is conjugated or oxidised to various inactive forms which are lost within a week. The conjugated forms, such as the β–glucuronide, are excreted *via* the bile and then lost in the faeces. Various polar and chain-shortened metabolites of retinoic acid are mainly excreted in the urine.

Toxicity

Toxicity due to vitamin A is referred to as hypervitaminosis A. Vitamin A is toxic in excessive amounts, whereas carotene is not. A single dose of vitamin A around 200,000 μg given under medical supervision, should not produce toxic effects. Doses of 500,000 μg or more may produce toxic effects in some individuals which take a few days to clear up. The toxic effects produced by a single dose of about 10,000,000 μg (that is 10 grams of vitamin A) produces serious toxicity that may take several weeks to clear up. The main symptoms of acute toxicity (which is rare) include loss of appetite, nausea, vomiting, muscular weakness, nosebleeds, irritability, drowsiness, headaches, blurred vision (or diplopia), increased pressure of the cerebrospinal fluid, and peeling of the skin. In some laboratory animals, the bones may become very brittle.

Continuous intake of excessive amount of vitamin A over several months or years may also produce (chronic) toxicity. In such cases, the daily doses are generally less than about 100,000 μg and can occasionally be as low as 25,000 μg. The symptoms of chronic toxicity include itchiness, pigmentation and drying of the skin, bleeding gums, loss of appetite, weight loss, general weakness, stiffness and bone swellings, loss of hair, enlargement of the liver and spleen, blood disorders, occasionally blurred vision, and tenderness particularly around the long bones. Also, there may be abnormal skeletal development in children. These symptoms generally disappear after few weeks of vitamin A restriction.

Supplements of vitamin A are still measured in international units

(IU). 1 IU of vitamin A is equivalent to 0.3 microgram (μg) of retinol, and 1 μg of retinol is equivalent to 3.33 IU of vitamin A. It is generally considered that doses of vitamin A up to 10,000 IU (3,000 μg) per day are safe for adults. It is now believed that symptoms of vitamin A toxicity develop only when the capacity of the liver protein called apo-retinol-binding protein is exceeded. Massive doses of vitamin A derivatives have been used in clinical trials on some forms of cancer.

High doses of provitamin A carotenoids alone do not cause toxicity because conversion of carotenoids to vitamin A is regulated by the body to maintain an optimum level of the vitamin. Overdoses of β–carotene do not appear to be toxic but can produce a yellowing of the skin as a side effect. This was at one time hailed as an alternative to getting a suntan. This practice cannot be recommended because large doses are required to produce the effect and also possible long term effects have not been fully investigated. Anyway, it is generally agreed that an unnatural looking tan develops.

Deficiency

There are a number of very obvious signs of vitamin A deficiency, and most of these refer to the eyes. At the outset, before considering these signs, it is worth explaining a number of medical terms which are used in this area. Xerosis is essentially any excessive dryness and it may be divided into xeroderma and xerophthalmia. Xeroderma is an excessive dryness of the skin accompanied by diminished cutaneous secretion and often a coarse buildup of the surface layers termed keratinisation. Keratinisation of the epidermis (or outer layer of skin) may result in desquamation or the shedding of the skin in scales. Xerothalmia is extreme dryness of the conjunctiva, which is the mucous membrane covering the surface of the eyeball and lining the eyelids. This condition may lead to inflammation (conjunctivitis) and the eyeball appears dull and opaque and loses its lustre. Bitot's spots are a useful clinical sign of vitamin A deficiency, particularly in young children. They are small raised greyish-white spots which appear in the eyes at an early stage of deficiency. Keratomalacia is a more serious condition where dryness of the conjunctiva leads to ulceration of the cornea, which is the transparent tissue constituting the outer eyeball. This rapid leads to serious corneal scaring. Nyctalopia, or night blindness is the inability of the eyes to adjust to seeing in dark conditions.

Night blindness is a very early sign of vitamin A deficiency. In contrast, hemeralopia or day blindness, is the inability to see as distinctly in very bright light as in dim light. This is a much rarer and later sign of deficiency. Ultimately vitamin A deficiency can lead to permanent blindness due to a combination of factors such as severe eye damage and deterioration of the optic nerve in some cases. Many children around three years of age in developing countries lose their sight each year because of vitamin A deficiency.

The symptoms of vitamin A deficiency in increasing order of severity include night blindness, dryness of the eyes, Bitot's spots, ulceration, scaring and eventual total blindness. Dryness of the akin occasionally leads to a scaly dermatitis. In chronic deficiency, especially in children who are most at risk, severe growth retardation may result and bone abnormalities may become evident. Damage to a number of systems may occur in severe cases. There may be an increased pressure in the cerebrospinal fluid in the brain. Nerve damage may lead to various disorders and contribute to blindness or deafness. Cysts may develop in various glands in the body. Some endocrine systems may be affected and sterility may result. A generalised debility and emaciation leads to increased risk of infections. Often kwashiorkor is a complicating factor. The senses may be dulled and taste, smell and appetite may be affected. Vitamin A is essential for spermatogenesis and regeneration of the visual pigment rhodopsin.

β–Carotene has a useful function of its own namely, its antioxidant capacity. The conjugated double bond system of this carotenoid is a powerful quencher of the single oxygen generated in immune response reactions. Therefore, malnourished children suffering from infection may not have enough antioxidant capacity needed to fight disease.

Some synthetic retinoids may exert an anti-tumour action, possibly by combining with cellular retinoic acid-binding protein. These substances generally have little or no vitamin A activity. So, it is possible that they may compete with active metabolites of vitamin A for certain growth promoting receptor sites and thus block their actions at the cellular level.

Retinol and ethanol (alcohol) compete for the enzyme alcohol dehydrogenase in various tissues. The activity of this enzyme is essential for converting retinol to retinal, the active visual form. Alcohol therefore impairs utilisation of vitamin A and may lead to night blindness in chronic alcoholics.

The symptoms of vitamin A deficiency are similar in most animals. However, in cattle (but not in humans), β–carotene has some functions that are unrelated to its potential to form vitamin A. Lack of β–carotene causes a variety of reproductive disorders and even abortions in cattle. The butterfat content of the milk is decreased and calves have a decreased vitality. It seems that while β–carotene can be converted to vitamin A; the reverse does not occur.

Table 58.1. Relative biopotency of different forms of Vitamin A.

NAME	NOMINAL VALUE (percent)
all-trans Forms	
Retinol	100
Retinal	90 (theoretically 100)
Retinoic acid	about 65, but incomplete
3-Dehydroretinol	40
5,6-Epoxyretinoic acid	incomplete
Various cis forms	
mono-*cis Forms*	
13'-*cis*-Retinol	75
11'-*cis*-Retinol	24
9'-*cis*-Retinol	23
13'-*cis*-Retinal	93
11'-*cis*-Retinal	48
9'-*cis*-Retinal	19
13'-*cis*-Retinoic acid	4
9'-*cis*-Retinoic acid	1
di-cis Forms	
5',7'-*di-cis*-Retinol	15
3',7'-*di-cis*-Retinol	24
9',13'-*di-cis*-Retinol	24
11',13'-*di-cis*-Retinol	15
11',13'-*di-cis*-Retinal	31
9',13'-*di-cis*-Retinal	17

Table 58.2. Relative biopotency of some esters of vitamin A

NAME	NOMINAL VALUE (percent)
Retinol	100
Retinyl acetate	87
Retinyl phosphate	78
Retinyl β–glucuronide	60
Retinyl palmitate	55
13'-cis-Retinyl acetate, propionate	76
9'-cis-Retinyl acetate, propionate	19
9',13'-di-cis-Retinyl acetate, propionate	16

Some values given above are theoretical optimum values.

The values given are for the all-*trans* forms. The esters (either as storage or supplementary forms) of vitamin A have a relatively lower biological activity per unit mass because of the additional group linked to the active retinol moiety.

Esters of retinoic acid are termed retinoyl esters. For example, the conjugated form, retinoyl β–glucuronide, is an inactive excretory product found in bile.

Table 58.3. Relative biopotency of different carotenoids

NAME	NOMINAL VALUE (percent)	
all-*trans*-Retinol [1]	100	
Provitamin A carotenoids *all-trans Forms*		
β–Carotene	50, or less	
Cryptoxanthin	28	
α–Carotene	26	average value 24 *
β–Zeacarotene	25	
γ–Carotene	21	
Various cis forms *of the above carotenoids*		
mono-*cis* Forms	16 − 7	
di-*cis* Forms	trace	
Other carotenoids		
Lutein, Zeaxanthin, *meso*-Zeaxanthin, Lycopene	0	

1. all-*trans*-Retinol is taken as a standard at 100 percent.

* Apart from β–carotene, the other provitamin A carotenoids on average, may be taken to have a relative activity of 24.

Table 58.4. Retinol activity equivalents (RAE) * associated with vitamin A and provitamin A compounds in the human.

COMPOUND	AMOUNT (µg giving 1 µg RAE)	RELATIVE BIOPOTENCY
all-*trans*-Retinol	1	1/1
all-*trans*-β-Carotene in oil	2	1/2
all-*trans*-β-Carotene in food	12	1/12
Other Provitamin A Carotenoids		
α–Carotene	24	1/24
γ–Carotene	24	1/24
β-Zeacarotene	24	1/24
β–Cryptoxanthin	24	1/24

* To be distinguished from retinol equivalents (RE) which are inaccurate. Since 2001, RE has been replaced by RAE.

Table 58.5. Relative biopotency of some Vitamin A and carotenoid compounds in the human (all values given as retinol activity equivalents, RAE, per 100 micrograms)

NAME	NOMINAL VALUE (RAE per 100 µg)
Retinol	100
Retinol acetate	87
Retinol palmitate	55
β–Carotene	8.3
Other provitamin A Carotenoids (e.g., α–Carotene, γ–Carotene, β-Cryptoxanthin and β-Zeacarotene)	4.2
All other Carotenoids	0

Table 58.6. Conversion of β–carotene to vitamin A by various animals

Species	PERCENT OF β–CAROTENE CONVERTED TO VITAMIN A	RATIO
Rat	50	2 : 1
Poultry	50	2 : 1
Dog	27	4 : 1
Horse	17	6 : 1
Swine	15	7 : 1
Sheep	15 – 12	7 : 1 – 8 : 1
Cattle	12	8 : 1
Fox	8	12 : 1
Cat	0	not utilised
Mink	0	not utilised

Table 58.7. Vitamin A compendium

FOOD GROUP	VITAMIN A LEVEL
Milk / Products	Very low / Medium
Eggs	Low
Meat and fish	Very variable
Fats and oils	Very variable
Grain and products	Nil
Nuts and pulses	Low
Root vegetables	Medium, variable
Leaf vegetables	Medium, variable
Fruit	Medium, variable
Sweets	Nil

The levels include the contribution of various provitamin A carotenoids.

59

Vitamin K (and Coenzyme Q$_{10}$)

Common Name

Vitamin K.

Alternative names

Blood coagulation factor. Koagulation vitamin.
Antihaemorrhagic vitamin or factor. Prothrombin factor.
The K Group. K$_1$, K$_2$, K$_3$.
Menaquinone. Phylloquinone. Phytonadione.
Phytyl- or phyto- menadione. naphthoquinone,
Alpha- and beta- phylloquinone. Farnoquinone.
Menadione. Menaphytone. Prenylmenaquinone.

Some of the above terms are obsolete.

History

1929: Dam observed the slow clotting of blood in chickens on fat-free diets.

1934: Dam and Schønheyder named the missing factor in synthetic diets Vitamin K (K being the first letter of the German word Koagulation and fortuitously the next letter free at that time).

1935: Almquist and Stokstad demonstrate Vitamin K in alfalfa and fish meal.

1939: Dam and Karrer isolated Vitamin K from alfalfa. Doisy, *et al.*, showed that the vitamin from alfalfa was one form, K$_1$, whereas McKee, *et al.*, isolated Vitamin K$_2$ from fishmeal. In the same year, McCorquodale, *et al.*, determined the structure of K$_1$, Almquist and

Klose reported the antihaemorrhagic activity of the vitamin and Fieser synthesised it.

1943: Dam and Doisy were awarded the Nobel Prize for their work on vitamin K.

1957: The coenzyme, CoQ_{10}, was discovered. This coenzyme, although not a vitamin, has a structural resemblance to both Vitamin K and Vitamin E which are quinone derivatives. Ubiquinone is another name for CoQ_{10}.

1974: The function of vitamin K in converting glutamate residues to γ–carboxyglutamate in prothrombin was discovered.

1994: Thijssen and Drittij-Reijnders discovered that vitamin K_1 can be converted into some vitamin K_2 in the body.

-----: Apart from derivatives, no further fat-soluble Vitamins have been discovered to date. Therefore, there are only four fat-soluble vitamins, namely Vitamins A, D, E and K, respectively.

----- : Vitamin K is now a generic term for menadione and all its derivatives that exhibit qualitatively the biological activity of phylloquinone (K_1).

Nature

Vitamin K has two natural vitamers, vitamin K_1 and vitamin K_2, and three synthetic vitamers K_3, K_4 and K_5.

Vitamin K_1 (phylloquinone) is a plant source of vitamin K found in fruit and vegetables. Vitamin K_1 exists naturally as the active 2'-*trans*-isomer. However, biological samples may also contain some inactive cis-isomer. In animals, phylloquinone is found in liver and heart, but is only present at low concentrations in the brain. When vitamin K_1 is absorbed, it goes mainly to the liver and stays there. It has a relatively short half-life.

Vitamin K_2 (menaquinone or MK) is a bacterial source of vitamin K.

Vitamin K_2 has a polyisoprenoid unsaturated side-chain of various lengths up to 13 isoprene units. These compounds are called menaquinones-n, or MK-n, where n is the number of isoprene units. The majority of homologues have from n=6 to n=9 and make up about 90% of the total menaquinones in bacteria. In animals, menaquinones (mainly MK-4) are present at higher concentrations (compared to phylloquinone) in the pancreas, salivary gland and brain. This MK-4 accumulation in non-hepatic tissues is likely a result of synthesis rather than uptake from the gut. MK-7 is ten times better absorbed than vitamin K_1; only 10 percent of vitamin K_1 is absorbed from green leafy vegetables. Vitamin K_2 also goes to the liver, but from there it is redistributed by low density lipoproteins.

Vitamin K_2 activates a protein called vitamin K-dependent matrix γ–carboxyglutamic acid protein (MGP) which is a potent inhibitor of calcification. MGP and osteocalcin are both calcium-binding proteins that may participate in the organisation of bone tissue. Vitamin K_2 may help prevent arterial calcification and thus may lower the risk of cardiovascular disease.

Vitamin K_3 (menadione or 2-methyl-1,4-naphthoquinone) is toxic in large doses and can cause allergic reactions, haemolytic anaemia and cytotoxicity in liver cells. Menadione can be alkylated to yield K_2 vitamers (menaquinones, MK-n, n=1-13) in the body, so it may be considered as a provitamin. Menadione is alkylated at position 2 with an isoprenoid side-chain in the liver and then it has the same activity as phylloquinone.

Vitamin K_4 (menadiol or 2-methyl-1,4-naphthohydroquinone) induces mutations in the Escherichia coli enzyme nitrate reductase A and has recently been reported to have inhibitory effects on prostate cancer.

Vitamin K_5 (synkamin or 2-methyl-4-amino-1-naphthol) is used in the pet food industry to inhibit fungal growth and can mimic the effect of insulin. Vitamins K_2, K_3 and K_5 have been found to exert antitumor effects.

Chemically speaking, all vitamin K compounds are polyisoprenoid substituted derivatives of 2-methyl-1,4-naphtoquinone. They are synthesised in higher plants and by many microorganisms including many that live in the gut. The gut bacteria contribute significantly to the daily intake of vitamin K in humans. The term vitamin K is now used as a generic descriptor for menadione and all of its derivatives with phylloquinone activity.

The plant forms of vitamin K comprise the vitamin K_1 series, which are all phylloquinones. The bacterial forms of vitamin K comprise the vitamin K_2 series, which are all menaquinones. Menadione derivatives comprise the synthetic vitamin K series, K_3, K_4 and K_5. Phylloquinone is usually taken as the most representative form of the vitamin K group, although menadione may be considered as the parent compound.

All the naturally occurring forms of vitamin K (the K_1 and the K_2 series) are lipid-soluble. The gut bacteria can convert K_1 into K_2. Vitamin K_2 is the main storage form in animals. The number of 5-carbon isoprenoid units in a substituted side chain is usually specified when considering a particular derivative. Although substitution can occur in the human body, compounds with initially shorter side chains have relatively higher potencies on a weight basis. Menadione itself is without an isoprenoid side chain and only becomes active after it has been converted (alkylated) to one of the menaquinones. Yet, it is the most potent form of vitamin K. The relative biopotencies of various forms of vitamin K are given in Table 59.1. The most representative and common phylloquinone has 20 carbon atoms (or 4 isoprenoid units, of which only the first one has a double bond) in its side chain. It has a nominal biopotency of 100, which gives menadione a value of 230. The menaquinones are more variable and can have from 4 to 13 isoprenoid units (each of which contains a double bond), or from 20 up to 55 carbon atoms in the side chain. The most commonly occurring of these menaquinone compounds are those containing 6, 7, or 9 isoprenoid units. Taking an average figure for these, the nominal biopotency of dietary menaquinones is usually taken as 75. Some derivatives of menadione are water-soluble. Vitamin K is a relatively stable vitamin.

Biological Functions

- Vitamin K regulates the plasma concentration of several blood coagulation proteins. These clotting factors are termed factor VII (or proconvertin), factor IX (or plasma thromboplastin component, or occasionally Christmas factor), factor X (or Stuart-Prower factor), and factor II (or prothrombin), respectively. All of these factors are synthesised in the liver but each requires vitamin K to be converted to the active form. In each case the activation process involves a modification of glutamic acid residues which are changed to γ–carboxyglutamic acid residues. Chemically the change involves adding an extra carboxyl group to the non-attached carboxyl end of glutamic acid, thus generating a novel amino acid in what is termed a post-translational modification. In other words, the change occurs after the protein has been synthesised. It is now known that the double carboxyl terminal can combine with calcium to form a chelate of the form $(Ca^{++})(COO^-)_2$. It is this property which is essential to the clotting function of these factors. In the absence of any one of these factors the clotting mechanism becomes defective. This is because each factor depends on at least one other factor in a complicated series of events which ultimately catalyses the conversion of fibrinogen to fibrin to form a blood clot.

- Vitamin K cooperates with a specific microsomal enzyme called vitamin K-dependent carboxylase to carry out the conversion of glutamic acid to the γ–carboxyl form in the presence of carbon dioxide and other factors. The microsomes are essentially membrane components in the cell that can be isolated using special techniques. The only clearly defined role of vitamin K in the human is in the control of blood clotting. Vitamin K has been used therapeutically to prevent haemorrhage in a number of conditions, for example before surgery and even to ease heavy menstrual bleeding.

• A so-called vitamin K cycle also occurs in liver microsomes but its role is not fully understood at present. One theory is that during carboxylation the vitamin must be converted to its hydroquinone form, which in turn must be converted to the 2,3-epoxide form before being recycled back to the main quinone form. Apart from the enzyme carboxylase, which seems to be dependent on the hydroquinone form, other enzymes are also involved. The conversion of the hydroquinone to the epoxide form (occasionally termed oxide) requires the action of the monooxygenase enzyme. The epoxide may be converted back to the quinone form by the action of an epoxide reductase enzyme. This last step in particular is sensitive to the action of various coumarin antagonists. These substances, such as warfarin, thus block the activity of vitamin K and lead to symptoms of vitamin K deficiency.

• It has been discovered that clotting factors are not the only proteins that vitamin K can act on. Several other proteins containing γ–carboxyglutamic acid residues have been found in different tissues in the body. It appears that a number of proteins contain a common sequence of amino acids containing some glutamic acid residues and that these residues can also be carboxylated in the presence of vitamin K. The function of these proteins is largely unknown at the present time. Some of these proteins are found in plasma, bone, kidney, aorta, tendon, lung, spleen, pancreas and placenta, but species differences are considerable.

• A calcium-binding protein called osteocalcin, which contains γ–carboxyglutamic acid is found in bone. Vitamin K, particularly K_2, functions as a cofactor for the enzyme that catalyzes the carboxylation of osteocalcin and may help protect against osteoporosis by collaborating with vitamin D.

• Some ribosomal proteins have also been found to contain γ–carboxyglutamic acid. The amino acid has also been found in plaque deposits resulting from atherosclerosis. In many cases, it appears that these proteins are involved in aspects of calcium metabolism.

- It has frequently been suggested that vitamin K may be involved in electron transport and oxidative phosphorylation, although it is now generally accepted that the actual carrier involved is a close relative of vitamin K namely, ubiquinone.

- Some studies have indicated that Vitamin K may offer some protection against bone fractures and cancers.

- Vitamin K, particularly K_2, functions as a cofactor for the enzyme that catalyzes the carboxylation of osteocalcin and may help protect against osteoporosis by collaborating with vitamin D.

Requirement

In general, the absorption and excretion of vitamin K is similar to that of vitamin E. But unlike vitamin E, vitamin K is not stored to any extent in the body, although traces are found in the liver particularly after a meal. The phylloquinones and the menaquinones require bile salts to be absorbed in association with lipids via the lymph. A number of synthetic menadiones are water soluble and can be absorbed directly into the blood without the need for bile. Bean shoots, particularly alfalfa, are very rich sources of vitamin K. Other good sources include dark green vegetables, liver, fruit and some seed grains. The vitamin K compendium gives further details on dietary sources of the vitamin (Table 59.2). The recommended adult daily intake of vitamin K in males is 120 μg/d and in females is 90 μg/d, respectively. An additional requirement during pregnancy or lactation is not specified; it is assumed that the general values given for adult women are sufficient.

The precise contribution of bacterially synthesized vitamin K_2 to human vitamin K requirement is largely unknown. Under normal dietary conditions, it appears that about half of the vitamin K requirement comes from vitamin K_1 in the diet while the other half is provided by vitamin K_2 from the gut bacteria. But it has also been suggested that the gut bacteria in healthy persons may be capable of providing all the vitamin K that they need. Mineral oils such as liquid paraffin in the diet (which is often used as a mild laxative) tend to decrease the absorption of vitamin K and also all the other fat-soluble vitamins. The level of the 2,3-epoxide form of the vitamin is increased following treatment with some coumarins. Warfarin accelerates the urinary excretion of vitamin K while reducing the loss in the faeces. A number of excretory metabolites of vitamin K, such as the conjugated □-glucuronide forms, have been postulated, and are under investigation at present.

Toxicity

Natural forms of vitamin K are non-toxic. In fact, vitamin K has even been used as a natural food preservative in much the same way as vitamins C and E. However, doses of synthetic (water soluble) vitamin K greater the 50 mg per day are not recommended. Excessive vitamin K in the form of menadione has produced kernicterus in low-weight babies due to haemolysis. Kernicterus is a neurological syndrome caused by damage to the basal ganglia and other nerve structures in the brain. It is due to bilirubin which arises from excessive breakdown of red blood cells during haemolytic jaundice. The bilirubin (which causes the yellow colour of jaundice) can enter the brain and become deposited in certain areas thus damaging them. In infants, the risk is greater because the liver may not be sufficiently developed to handle large amounts of bilirubin. Massive doses of vitamin K may also damage the liver. Menadione may react with sulfhydryl groups (–SH) and may inactivate certain enzymes or impair protein structures. In most perinatal conditions, especially, vitamin K_1 is a safer alternative to use.

Deficiency

In the healthy human, vitamin K deficiency is rare, because the gut bacteria are able to provide the bulk of the requirement. However, after treatment with certain antibiotics, such as sulphonamide, after certain operations and during some forms of biliary obstruction (obstructive jaundice), a deficiency can develop. A deficiency of vitamin K may occur during any condition which decreases lipid absorption such as sprue or steatorrhoea. Human infants may be deficient in vitamin K at birth. The observation that about 1 percent of infants are deficient vitamin K for the first week after birth, at a time when their gut bacteria has not yet been established, indicates that some additional vitamin K may be beneficial during pregnancy and lactation, but no such value has been set. Human milk is very poor in vitamin K. So, if an infant is found deficient, a single intramuscular injection of vitamin K may be indicated to prevent haemorrhagic disease. An alternative prophylactic measure is the administration of vitamin K to the mother shortly before birth, but this practice is less satisfactory.

Vitamin K deficiency results in prolonged clotting times which may lead to bleeding, shock and ultimately death in extreme cases. During vitamin K deficiency, there is a decrease in the plasma concentration of four blood clotting factors. The sequence of events is as follows. Factor VII is the first to decrease and this occurs rapidly. Factors IX, X, and II then decrease in that order but somewhat more slowly. Interestingly, the coumarins (anticoagulant drugs such as 4-hydroxycoumarin and warfarin) are known to suppress the vitamin K-dependent clotting factors competitively in the same order. Patients on treatment with anticoagulants should be carefully monitored as the duration of action of different drugs can vary. Vitamin K may be used as an antidote for such drugs in certain cases.

Birds are particularly susceptible to vitamin K deficiency, which leads to various haemorrhages if not corrected. Occasionally, pigs also run the risk of deficiency, particularly if maintained on certain high-moisture grain diets.

Coenzyme Q_{10}

Coenzyme Q_{10} is chemically similar to vitamin K although it is not a vitamin. Coenzyme Q_{10} can be produced naturally and is found in every cell in the body. The coenzyme can exist in three oxidation states; a fully oxidised state called Coenzyme Q_{10} (CoQ_{10}), a partially reduced radical state called semiquinone ($CoQ_{10}H\cdot$) and a fully reduced state called ubiquinol ($CoQ_{10}H_2$). Ubiquinone contains a polyprenylated side-chain which is ten units long in mammals. The reduced ubiquinol form has been shown to be more effectively absorbed than ubiquinone. Ubiquinol is converted to ubiquinone and *vice versa* while carrying out its function. Either form can be reduced or oxidized to form the other. Young people can easily convert ubiquinone to ubiquinol but in older people less of this conversion occurs. Also, people who take statins have reduced levels of ubiquinone. It is recommended that older people (many of whom are on statins) should take supplements of CoQ_{10}, preferably the reduced form. Ubiquinol is involved with the electron transport chain where it forms a complex with cytochrome c oxidoreductase (called Complex III) during the production of ATP in the mitochondria. Ubiquinol is also a potent antioxidant. It assists in maintaining the normal oxidative state of low-density lipoprotein (LDL). High doses of ubiquinone, because of its similarity to vitamin K, may decrease the anticoagulant effect of warfarin. Low levels of CoQ_{10} may contribute to fatigue. Decreased levels of CoQ_{10} are associated with a number of diseases and are under intense study at the present time.

Table 59.1. Relative biopotency of different forms of vitamin K

NAME	NOMINAL VALUE (percent)
Vitamin K_1 (plant phylloquinones [a])	100
Vitamin K_2 (bacterial and animal multiprenylmenaquinones [a])	75, average
Vitamin K_3 (synthetic menadiones)	230
Menadione sodium bisulphite complex [b]	84
Menadione dimethyl pyrimidinol bisulphite [b]	120
Menadione (provitamin, 2-methyl-1,4-naphthoquinone)	0

a. Generally, isoprenologs with 3 to 5 isoprenoid groups in either phylloquinone or menaquinone compounds have maximum biological activity. As the polyisoprene side-chain gets longer the biopotency decreases.

b. Water-soluble forms of vitamin K.

Table 59.2. Vitamin K compendium

FOOD GROUP	VITAMIN K LEVEL
Milk and products	Very low
Eggs	Low
Meat and fish	Very variable
Fats and oils	Medium, variable
Grain and products	Medium
Nuts and pulses	High, variable
Root vegetables	Very low
Leaf vegetables	Very high, variable
Fruit	Very low
Sweets	Nil

60

Vitamin D

Common name

Vitamin D.

Alternative names

Vitamin D_2 (plant origin). Ergocalciferol. Ercalciol.
Activated ergosterol. Calciferol. Oleovitamin D_2. Viosterol.
Vitamin D_3 (animal origin). Cholecalciferol. Calciol.
Activated 7-dehydrocholesterol. Oleovitamin D_3
D_2, D_3, D_4, D_5, D_6, D_7.
25-Hydroxy-D_3. Calcidiol.
1-alpha-25-dihydroxy-D_3. Calcitriol.
24,23-dihydroxy-D_3.
The D vitamins. D Group.
The sunshine vitamin.

Some of the above terms are obsolete, others refer to specific metabolites.

History

-----: Ancient peoples all over the world knew that some ailments could be healed by sunlight.

1645: Whistler wrote a thesis on "The English Disease".

1650: Glisson gave the first detailed description of the disease, now called rickets.

1815: Loebel cured the sick by exposing them to sunlight.

circa 1870: Cod liver oil was introduced as a regular cure for rickets,

154

and other ailments.

circa 1890: Palm associated rickets with the lack of sunlight.

circa 1893: Finsen conducted experiments with different sources of light and distinguished some of the different effects produced at different wavelengths.

1915: Mellanby found that animal fat (believed at that time to contain only Vitamin A), protected against rickets.

1918: Mellanby produced rickets in dogs on a restricted diet.

1919: Huldschinsky ameliorated rickets in children with ultraviolet light.

1922: Hess showed that liver oil contained the same factor that sunlight produces. McCollum showed a connection between calcium deposition in rachitic rats and the cod liver oil factor.

1924: Steenbock showed that foods that have been exposed to irradiation also exhibit antirachitic properties.

1925: McCollum coined the term Vitamin D for the antirachitic factor. Three years earlier, McCollum predicted that there was a 'fourth vitamin' (distinct from the then known A, B and C), and which is fat-soluble like A. Hess and Weinstock showed that irradiated skin prevented rickets, confirming Huldschinskey's early work.

1930: Mellanby isolated Vitamin D from cod liver oil.

1931: Angus was the first to crystallise Vitamin D. It was soon realised that there were two forms of Vitamin D.

1932: The structure of Vitamin D_2 was determined simultaneously by Windaus and by Askew. Askew named it ergocalciferol.

1936: Windaus identified the structure of Vitamin D_3, which is called cholecalciferol.

1964: Norman, *et al.*, detected three metabolites of Vitamin D that were active in preventing rickets.

1968: The 25-hydroxy derivative of Vitamin D_3 was identified by Blunt, *et al.*

1969: Suda, *et al.*, identified the corresponding 25-hydroxy derivative of Vitamin D_2.

1971, *et seq.*: Calcitriol, the 1,25-dihydroxy derivative of vitamin D_3, was first identified by Holick. The structure of calcitriol was discovered and reported simultaneously by several laboratories including DeLuca's and Kodicek's. This is the most active metabolite and is synthesised in the kidney.

1972: DeLuca, *et al.*, established the structure of the 24,25-dihydroxy metabolite, another active form of vitamin D_3.

-----: The designation Vitamin D_1 is not used. Vitamin D is now a generic descriptor for all secosteroid derivatives that exhibit qualitatively the biological activity of cholecalciferol.

Nature

Vitamin D is a close relative of the steroid molecule called cholesterol. Strictly speaking, the term vitamin D is now used as a generic descriptor for all secosteroids with cholecalciferol activity. Cholecalciferol is usually taken as the most representative compound of the vitamin D group (although ergocalciferol has the same activity in the human body). One microgram of either ergocalciferol (vitamin D_2) or cholecalciferol (vitamin D_3) has 40 international units of vitamin D activity. Vitamin D occurs in plants and animals. The main form in higher plants and microorganisms is derived from the provitamin ergosterol by photolysis (activation in the presence of ultraviolet light) to yield ergocalciferol, or vitamin D_2. The main animal form is derived also by photolysis from the provitamin 7-dehydrocholesterol to yield cholecalciferol, or vitamin D_3. In both cases photolysis causes ring opening (at the B ring), which activates the molecule and enables it to participate in hydroxylation reactions yielding even more active metabolites of vitamin D in the body. Normally the provitamins (which are similar to cholesterol) consist of four fused rings, labelled A, B, C and D, respectively, and a side chain which is attached to ring D. Different forms of vitamin D are listed in Table 60.1.

The relative biopotencies of a number of vitamin D compounds are given in Table 60.2. Alternative names for several vitamin D derivatives are given in Table 60.3. The only chemical difference between vitamin D_2 and vitamin D_3 occurs in the side chain attached to the D-ring. In the vitamin D_2 series, this side chain contains 9 carbon atoms and has an extra methyl group and one double bond. In the vitamin D_3 series, the side chain has only 8 carbon atoms and no double bond. The hydroxy derivatives of vitamin D_2 are believed to have similar activities to those of vitamin D_3 derivatives in the human. But to date most of the research on hydroxylated derivatives has been carried out on the vitamin D_3 series. It should be noted however that the D_2 and D_3 derivatives do not have equivalent activities in all animals studied, which is somewhat similar to the observations of β–carotene activity in different species. Hydroxyls in position 1 occur on the A ring, whereas hydroxyls in positions 24, 25 and 26 all occur on the side chain attached to ring D.

The main effects of vitamin D involve maintaining the levels of calcium and phosphate in the blood plasma by acting at various sites in the body including the gut, the bones and the kidneys. Vitamin D acts in conjunction with the parathyroid hormone, and is itself now considered as a hormone. Various derivatives of vitamin D do not all have the same quantitative or even qualitative effects at each site of action. Hence the relative biopotencies depend exactly on the effect and the site used for comparison. The overall values quoted in Table 60.2 are only approximate and subject to revision, and for some derivatives conceal an incompleteness of biological activity. Further details on specific functions of each derivative are given in the following text.

Many chemical analogues of vitamin D are under investigation at the present time. Some of these promote bone calcium mobilization or intestinal calcium absorption or both, while others act as antagonists. Vitamin D is a very stable vitamin. Because there are several active metabolites of vitamin D, each with a specific range of functions, it is necessary to have some knowledge of the metabolism of the vitamin for a proper understanding of its various functions. The overall picture of vitamin D metabolism is summarised in Figure 60.1.

Figure 60.1. General pathways of vitamin D metabolism

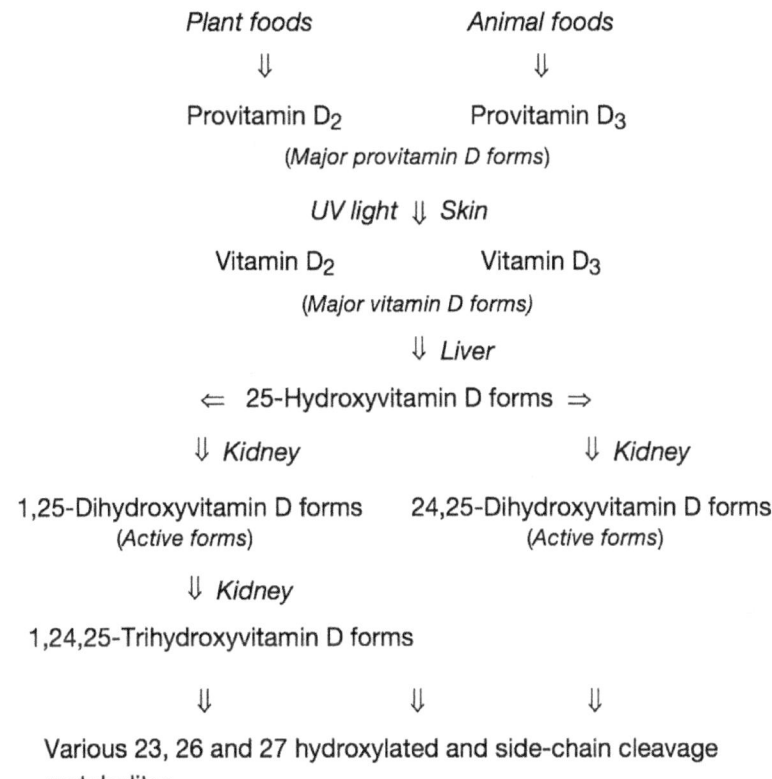

Plant foods   Animal foods

⇓   ⇓

Provitamin D_2 Provitamin D_3

(*Major provitamin D forms*)

UV light ⇓ *Skin*

Vitamin D_2 Vitamin D_3

(*Major vitamin D forms*)

⇓ *Liver*

⇐ 25-Hydroxyvitamin D forms ⇒

⇓ *Kidney*   ⇓ *Kidney*

1,25-Dihydroxyvitamin D forms   24,25-Dihydroxyvitamin D forms

(*Active forms*)   (*Active forms*)

⇓ *Kidney*

1,24,25-Trihydroxyvitamin D forms

⇓   ⇓   ⇓

Various 23, 26 and 27 hydroxylated and side-chain cleavage metabolites

(*Mostly inactive forms and a wide variety of lactones, oxo derivatives and acidic derivatives such as calcitroic acid excreted mainly in the bile and lost in the faeces*)

In recent years, some of the active metabolites of vitamin D have been given special names for convenience. The terms calciol (vitamin D_3) calcidiol (25-hydroxyvitamin D_3), and calcitriol (1,25-dihydroxyvitamin D_3), are generally used.

Biological Functions

• Like other steroids, vitamin D in the blood plasma is protein bound. All the hydroxy metabolites of D_2 and D_3 appear to be transported on the same carrier protein called transcalciferin or vitamin D-binding protein. The 25-hydroxy and the 24,25-dihydroxy forms are tightly bound whereas the 1,25-dihydroxy and the parent vitamin D forms are more loosely bound. The vitamin itself is stored mainly in adipose tissue but at a lower concentration than in the plasma. Some vitamin D is also stored in the liver and the skin. The $25(OH)D_3$ metabolite, calcidiol, is stored mainly in muscle and consequently is a major storage form in the body.

• The half-life of calcidiol in blood plasma is about 3 weeks in normal individuals but it can be up to twice as long in patients with kidney failure. The half-life of 24-hydroxycalcidiol is about the same. However, vitamin D itself is rapidly cleared by the liver or stored in adipose tissue. Calcitriol also has a very short half-life which is only a few hours at most.

• Vitamin D cooperates closely with several hormones in regulating calcium and phosphate levels in the body. The main hormones include the parathyroid hormone (or parathormone) and a thyroid hormone called calcitonin, although the growth hormone of the pituitary gland, insulin and prostaglandin E_2 are also involved. Certain steroid hormones including the glucocorticoids of the adrenal glands and estrogens also have effects on the calcium metabolism of bone. It is believed that relatively lower levels of the latter in older women may be a significant factor in the etiology of osteoporosis.

• The level of free calcium ions in the blood plasma regulates the secretion of the parathyroid hormone. Low calcium levels increase the secretion, whereas high levels inhibit the secretion of the hormone. Increased inorganic phosphate ion levels effectively neutralise calcium ions, thereby indirectly stimulate parathyroid hormone secretion. The parathyroid hormone itself has profound effects on calcium and phosphate metabolism.

Briefly, it promotes the absorption of both ions from the gut, it increases calcium (and phosphate) mobilisation from bone at high levels, while at lower levels it promotes bone formation, and it decreases calcium excretion but increases phosphate excretion by the kidney. The overall effect of the parathyroid hormone is to increase the calcium level but decrease the phosphate level in the blood.

- Calcitonin has the opposite effect to the parathyroid hormone regarding its action on bone calcium. Calcitonin is rapidly cleared by the kidney. It has a shorter duration of action on circulating plasma calcium than the parathyroid hormone but its initial effect occurs faster. And, it promotes calcium excretion by the kidney, while inhibiting the synthesis of calcitriol in that organ. Calcitonin also inhibits the resorption of bone collagen and consequently the excretion of hydroxyproline in the urine. All these effects are more potent in children than in adults. The overall effect of calcitonin is to decrease plasma calcium and phosphate levels. High doses of calcitonin may inhibit gastric secretion but they have a therapeutic use in certain cases of hypercalcemia. Although calcitonin acts as a sensitive fine control helping the parathyroid hormone and vitamin D to maintain calcium and phosphate levels, it is not strictly essential for life. The main effects of vitamin D, the parathyroid hormone and calcitonin in regulating calcium and phosphate metabolism are summarised in Table 60.4.

- Vitamin D_2 and D_3 have negligible biological activity *per se*. Only when they are converted to key hydroxylated derivatives can they exert their effects on calcium and phosphate metabolism. The concentrations of calcidiol, 24-hydroxycalcidiol and calcitriol in blood plasma are normally of the order 30, 0.03 and 0.03 µg per litre, respectively. In other words, the concentration of calcidiol is normally about one-thousand times greater than that of 24-hydroxycalcidiol or calcitriol. The concentrations of the latter metabolites are approximately the same when plasma calcium is in the normal range. It appears that there is a reciprocal relationship between the levels of these two metabolites which cooperate to restore the normal calcium level in the blood whenever it is disturbed. However, a number of other hormones, as we have seen in the previous section, are also involved in calcium homeostasis.

- The function of each of the more active metabolites of vitamin D will now be considered. It should be noted, however, that much work remains to be done to fully understand the role of each metabolite in the complicated vitamin D picture. As with all areas of rapidly advancing knowledge, some of the details may change with time.

- Calcidiol, 25(OH)D$_3$, is formed in the liver under the action of a microsomal enzyme called 25-hydroxylase. In high doses this metabolite is more potent than caicitriol in stimulating kidney resorption of calcium and phosphate. It may have a major role to play in regulating calcium fluxes and contractility in muscle where it is present in high concentrations. Unlike the parent vitamin D$_3$, calcidiol has some ability to act directly on gut and bone, but its duration of action is short. Under normal conditions, calcidiol is converted to calcitriol in the kidney. This step is strictly regulated by a number of factors including the levels of calcium and phosphate in the blood plasma, and is also under the influence of the parathyroid hormone.

- Calcitriol, 1,25(OH)$_2$D$_3$, is formed from calcidiol in the proximal tubules of the kidney by the action of a mitochondrial enzyme called 1-hydroxylase (or 1-α–hydroxylase). It is by far the most potent metabolite of vitamin D and acts very quickly. In contrast, there is a 12-hour delay before vitamin D itself exerts its effects in the body. Calcitriol functions as a hormone to regulate calcium and phosphate metabolism. It promotes calcium absorption from the gut. Specific receptors exist in the cytoplasm of several target tissues including the gut, bone, kidney and brain, that enable calcitriol to be transported and enter the nucleus. In this regard, there is a similarity to the hormone-like metabolite of vitamin A namely retinol which was considered in Chapter 58. The hormone-like activities of vitamin D may be summarised as follows. The vitamin is synthesised in the body (skin), although admittedly this process requires the presence of ultraviolet light. It is carried in the blood to various organs (such as liver, kidney and placenta) where it is activated. From these organs, activated metabolites travel again in the blood to other target tissues where they exert their biological effects. Finally, the levels of various active forms of vitamin D are subject to feed-back regulatory mechanisms.

- When calcitriol enters the nucleus of certain target tissues it stimulates the synthesis of RNA which in turn directs the synthesis of specific calcium binding proteins. In the intestinal epithelial cell, one specific type of calcium binding protein is formed, whereas, in other cells, a different type is synthesised. Calcitriol also promotes the absorption of phosphate from the intestine by a separate mechanism. It also appears to play a role in phospholipid metabolism in gut cell membranes. Some of the effects of calcitriol on phosphate metabolism may be independent of influence by the parathyroid hormone.

- Calcitriol promotes the reabsorption of bone and the elevation of blood plasma calcium. It is known that specialised bone cells regulate the flux of calcium and phosphate to and from the bone structure. Although essentially a solid structure, bone contains a significant fluid phase. It is believed that calcium in the bone fluid compartment is partially separated from the calcium in the external body fluid by a layer of cells, mainly osteoblasts. Osteoblasts generally promote bone mineralisation whereas other types of bone cells namely osteoclasts and osteocytes generally promote bone resorption. Calcitriol may promote differentiation of bone cells to give rise to osteoclasts. Apparently, the parathyroid hormone increases while calcitonin decreases the permeability of bone cells to calcium. The vitamin D3 metabolite calcitriol, on the other hand, promotes the active transport of calcium specifically from the osteoblasts into the surrounding extracellular fluid. However, the net movement of calcium to or from bone depends on several factors working together.

- Calcitriol also acts directly to stimulate the reabsorption of calcium by the kidney. The synthesis of calcitriol is regulated by the parathyroid hormone which stimulates the kidney enzyme involved in the 1-hydroxylation step. In turn, the release of the parathyroid hormone is stimulated by a fall in plasma calcium levels. On the other hand, a rise in plasma calcium inhibits the synthesis of calcitriol while stimulating the synthesis of 24,25-dihydroxyvitamin D_3 (24-hydroxy-calcidiol) instead. The level of phosphate in the plasma also appears to exert an effect on the kidney enzyme. Low levels stimulate the formation of calcitriol. A rise in the level of calcitriol itself inhibits its own further synthesis from calcidiol but stimulates the synthesis of 24-hydroxycalcidiol. In some cases, calcitriol may be synthesised in tissues other than the kidney, for example the placenta. In certain cancers and in sarcoidosis, calcitriol may also be synthesised in large amounts.

- The main functions of 24-hydroxycalcidiol, $24,25(OH)_2D_3$, appears to be the stimulation of normal bone formation rather than the resorption of calcium from bone. 24-Hydroxycalcidiol also stimulates calcium absorption by the intestine and promotes general growth. It is possible that a further metabolite of 24-hydroxycalcidiol namely 1,24,25-trihydroxyvitamin D_3 (or 24-hydroxycalcitriol) may be responsible for these effects. The physiological significance of 24-hydroxycalcidiol appears to lie in its ability to antagonise some of the effects of calcitriol. In particular, it acts as a break on the effect of calcitriol which tends to elevate blood plasma calcium levels. High levels of both calcium and phosphate inhibit the formation of calcitriol by the kidney but increase the formation of 24-hydroxycalcidiol. In general, 24-hydroxycalcidiol is less active than calcitriol and has incomplete activity. Many of the details outlined above regarding the hydroxy metabolites of vitamin D are still under investigation.

- Through its various forms and functions, vitamin D is of key importance in the regulation of body calcium and phosphate levels. In general, it ensures the proper growth of bones and teeth and assists the parathyroid hormone and calcitonin in maintaining normal plasma levels of both minerals. It ensures that adequate quantities of calcium and phosphate are absorbed from the diet. And, it also exerts a fine control on the kidney which tends to minimise the loss of calcium in the urine under normal circumstances.

• Ketone 250 is another compound related to vitamin D which naturally occurs in a wide variety of plants and fish liver oils. It has a potency of only 10 percent relative to vitamin D itself, but may contribute to the overall requirement in marginal circumstances.

• An analogue of vitamin D called dihydrotachysterol has negligible antirachitic activity but in high doses has a significant effect on the calcium resorption from bone. The analogue may therefore be used in the treatment of hypoparathyroidism (a condition where the activity of the parathyroid gland is inadequate) in some patients. It is now believed that this analogue undergoes 25-hydroxylation in the liver. Unlike the natural metabolite of vitamin D_3, namely calcidiol, this 25-OH form does not require the further 1-hydroxylation for its effect. Furthermore, the level of the metabolite is not subject to feed-back regulation by the liver or kidney and this has advantages in therapeutic applications. Dihydrotachysterol has a short duration of action but a very rapid onset. It has only one-fiftieth the potency of vitamin D_3 in promoting calcium absorption in the gut, but it has about three times its potency in promoting calcium resorption from bone.

Requirement

There is no dietary requirement for vitamin D in humans who are exposed to sunlight on a regular basis. However, in temperate and cool climates not only does heavy clothing cut down the surface area of skin which is exposed to sunlight, but also the number of sunshine hours per day may be insufficient to allow enough vitamin D to be formed in the body. This is especially true during the Winter months. The fact that vitamin D can be synthesised in the body and act as a prohormone of the sterol type confers on it the dignity of a true human hormone. In one study, it was found that some five times more vitamin D_3 than vitamin D_2 was present in the body, indicating that sunlight is the principle source of the vitamin. However, the colour of the skin influences the rate of synthesis of the vitamin. Dark-coloured skin is slower than fair-coloured skin to synthesise vitamin D. However, as considered above, this ability is strictly limited by the availability of sunlight. In other words, vitamin D should also be considered as a classical vitamin and essential nutrient in a nutritional context. In fact, the nutritional sources of vitamin D are very limited. The chief sources are various animal fats and oils and particularly fish liver oils. Some of the vitamin D is esterified in fish oils. Milk is also a good source of the vitamin, especially when it is fortified. Organ meats, eggs, butter and margarine are other good sources. The only relevant plant sources include a number of fungi and yeasts. However, some plants (and fish) contain ketone 250, a substance related to vitamin D which has some biological activity.

The compendium gives further details (Table 60.5). The absolute minimum intake of vitamin D required to prevent deficiency in adults not exposed to sunlight is probably about 2.5 µg per day. The recommended adult daily intake of vitamin D in both males and in females is 15 µg/d. Sedentary or housebound adults may require a higher intake. Similarly, dark-skinned people may require a slightly higher intake than fair-skinned people because of the effect of pigmentation in reducing the synthesis of vitamin D in skin exposed to sunlight. Some authors have suggested that elderly people may benefit from an increased intake of vitamin D to offset a decreased ability to absorb calcium from the diet or an increased tendency to reabsorb bone calcium. However, there is no general agreement on this point at present. Bile promotes the absorption of lipids in general and hence vitamin D from the gut. Inactive metabolites of vitamin are excreted also in the bile and lost in the faeces.

Toxicity

Vitamin D is potentially the most toxic of the vitamins. The toxicity due to vitamin D has been termed hypervitaminosis D. The acute toxic dose for adults is not known. However continuous intake of 2,500 µg per day for several months (or even 600 µg in some individuals) or even lower amounts, possible as low as 100 μg over more extended periods, have resulted in toxic symptoms. Doses as low as 50 μg per day in infants have also proved toxic. The acceptable daily intake in adults lies in the range 10 to 25 μg per day and the acceptable intake range for children lies in the range 5 to 10 μg per day.

Prolonged intake of over 20 μg vitamin D per day in children or adults produces demineralisation of bone, leading to fractures. Other toxic effects include increased blood plasma calcium levels particularly in infants, and nephrocalcinosis in children and adults. Nephrocalcinosis is characterised by generalised calcification in the kidneys caused by precipitation of calcium phosphates and calcium oxalates as stones. In general, the symptoms of toxicity include nausea, vomiting and loss of appetite resulting in a loss of weight. Increased thirst is a common symptom also, where the accompanying large intake of water increases the flow of urine. Gut disturbances, head pains (as distinct from headaches), depression and stupor may occur and in extreme cases extensive calcification of the kidney, lungs, heart and arteries may develop. In children, abnormal deposition of calcium in the bones also occurs, but in adults there may actually be a loss of calcium from the bones. The level of calcium in the circulating blood may be higher than normal but usually the level of phosphate remains normal. The level of calcidiol may be up to fifteen times higher than normal during hypervitaminosis D, but in contrast the level of calcitriol usually remains normal. The effect of high levels of vitamin D may be enhanced in certain diseases. Even under medical supervision, when patients are treated with vitamin D for certain diseases, there is a risk of toxicity, particularly when the treatment is prolonged. The treatment for vitamin D toxicity is to withdraw vitamin D and reduce calcium in the diet. More recently, treatment with calcitonin has proved useful in some cases of hypercalcemia.

Deficiency

Vitamin D deficiency is characterised by a fall in calcium and phosphate levels in the blood plasma and by an increased activity of the enzyme called alkaline phosphatase. In response to the fall in calcium, the parathyroid hormone levels are increased and bone resorption is accelerated. A marked reduction in the level of calcitriol also occurs. The solubility saturation point of calcium x phosphate has been estimated by Hebert, *et al.*, to be between 6.0 and 4.7 (mmol^2/l^2) *in vivo*. So, in theory, provided the calcium and phosphate levels (expressed as millimole per litre of blood plasma) maintain a value greater than this range, when multiplied together, rickets should not occur. But if this value falls below this range, rickets could possibly develop. Mild rickets is fairly common, even in Western countries. Deposition of minerals in newly formed bone fails to occur. In children, the collagenous matrix continues to grow, however, thus leading to soft bones, which easily bend to give such symptoms as bowlegs and other skeletal deformities. Rickets may be manifested by spinal curvature, poor posture (possibly as a result of muscular weakness in addition to skeletal deformities), bowlegs, knock-knees, soft bones, bone enlargements and other deformities. Sweating from the head may occur also. In children, also there may be inadequate tooth formation.

Adults whose bones have stopped growing do not develop rickets. Nevertheless, a deficiency of vitamin D in adults can have serious consequences resulting in osteomalacia. Osteomalacia is characterised by a loss of bone mass and a tendency for bones to fracture more easily. Bone pain is common and generalised muscle weakness may also develop as the deficiency progresses. Similar symptoms of deficiency occur in many animals. Hens with vitamin deficiency may lay eggs with thin shells. In all cases, unless vitamin D deficiency is treated, tetany results and ultimately death follows. Infants, in particular, are prone to develop tetany or convulsions at an early stage of deficiency.

Certain gut disorders tend to decrease the absorption of vitamin D from the diet. Liver and kidney disorders may also have profound effects on the proper utilisation of the vitamin in the body. Also, it has been discovered that a rare genetic disorder can result in a vitamin D-resistant form of rickets which occurs mainly in males and is characterised by a failure of the kidney to adequately reabsorb phosphate. In such cases, it has been found that normal levels of vitamin D and its metabolites in the body fail to maintain normal calcium or phosphate levels. Massive doses of calcidiol, however, may be used to treat the condition. Alcoholics tend to have lower levels of calcidiol than normal individuals but the implications of this finding are uncertain at present. Prolonged use of certain drugs such as barbiturates may increase the activity of microsomal enzymes in the liver and may accelerate the destruction of certain metabolites of vitamin D leading to the development of osteomalacia in individuals with an otherwise adequate intakes of vitamin D.

A surprisingly large number of children, even in Western countries, have inadequate intakes of vitamin D, often as low as 25 percent of the recommended level. Industrial city children, in particular, are at risk of developing rickets during periods of rapid growth. Although fortunately most children, even those with decreased calcidiol blood levels, never exhibit any symptoms. The observation that rickets and osteomalacia are more common in dark-skinned than in fair-skinned people who live in temperate climates cannot be fully explained by the differing rates of synthesis of vitamin D in the skin alone. Indeed, it has been found that the risk of developing vitamin D deficiency is almost invariably related to inadequate dietary intake rather than to the colour of the skin. In one study of Asians living in the UK, it was found that the dietary intake of vitamin was lower than in the general population. Also, the vitamin D status of pregnant Asian mothers was frequently low enough to cause osteomalacia, and the prevalence of rickets among their children was much higher. Clearly, in such cases, the age-old remedy, cod liver oil, would have proved beneficial.

Women who have repeated pregnancies also run the risk of developing calcium depletion which may be offset by increasing the intake of both calcium and vitamin D on a conservative basis. Older women are at greater risk of developing osteoporosis than older men. However, the origin of osteoporosis is far from clear and it is unlikely that simple supplementation with calcium or vitamin D can significantly prevent its development, which is believed to be related to hormonal changes rather that dietary deficiencies. In such cases, the best advice for the time being seems to be to remain physically active. Apart from maintaining general health and well-being, activity slows the rate of depletion of calcium from bone.

Table 60.1. Different forms of vitamin D.

VITAMIN	PRECURSOR
Vitamin D_2	Ergosterol
Vitamin D_3	7-Dehydrocholesterol
Vitamin D_4	22,23-Dihydroergosterol
Vitamin D_5	7-Dehydrositosterol
Vitamin D_6	7-Dehydrostigmasterol
Vitamin D_7	7-Dehydrocampesterol

The term vitamin D_1 is no longer used. Each active vitamin is formed by ultraviolet irradiation of its precursor. There are six main forms of vitamin D, each of which derives from a slightly different precursor. The difference between these precursors lies only in the composition of the side chain attached to ring D. Of all these forms, only the metabolites of vitamin D_2 and vitamin D_3 are of major nutritional importance in the human, although vitamin D_4 has only slightly less biological activity the them. A large number of derivatives of these compounds have some antirachitic activity and are under detailed investigation at the present time.

Table 60.2. Relative biopotency of different forms of Vitamin D

NAME	NOMINAL VALUE (percent)
Vitamin D_2 (Ergocalciferol; Ercalciol; plant form)	100
Vitamin D_3 (Cholecalciferol; Calciol; animal form)	100
25-Hydroxyvitamin D_3 (Calcidiol)	150
24,25-Dihydroxyvitamin D_3	qualitative differences
1,25-Dihydroxyvitamin D_3 (Calcitriol)	1,000 [a]
1,24,25-Trihydroxyvitamin D_3	qualitative differences
Ketone 250	10
Dihydrotachysterol	very weak

a. Estimates of the relative biopotency of 1,25-dihydroxyvitamin D_3 vary from around 500 to as high as 1,500.

The hydroxy derivatives of vitamin D_2 are thought to have similar activities to those of vitamin D_3 in the human. Various 26-hydroxy forms also occur, but are now believed to be partial breakdown products with little biological activity.

Alternative names for some of the above compounds are given in Table 60.3.

Table 60.3. Alternative names for key forms of vitamin D and its derivatives

VITAMIN or DERIVATIVE	ALTERNATIVE NAMES	ABBREVIATION
Vitamin D_1 *	------	------
Vitamin D_2	Ergocalciferol, Ercalciol	D_2
Vitamin D_3	Cholecalciferol [a], Calciol	D_3
25-Hydroxyvitamin D_3	Calcifediol, Calcidiol	$25(OH)D_3$
1,25-Dihydroxyvitamin D_3	Calcitriol	$1,25(OH)_2D_3$
24,25-Dihydroxyvitamin D_3	24Hydroxycalcidiol	$24,25(OH)_2D_3$
1,24,25-Trihydroxyvitamin D_3	1-Hydroxycalcitriol	$1,24,25(OH)_3D_3$

* The term vitamin D_1 is no longer used.

a. 1 µg cholecalciferol = 40 international units of vitamin D.

Table 60.4. Comparison of the effects of vitamin D, the parathyroid hormone and calcitonin, on calcium and phosphate metabolism in the body

SITE OF ACTION	VITAMIN D	PARATHYROID HORMONE	CALCITONIN
Intestine	Increases calcium and phosphate absorption (mainly as calcitriol).	Increases calcium and phosphate absorption (by stimulating calcitriol synthesis).	Decreases calcium and phosphate absorption (by inhibiting calcitriol synthesis).
Bone	Increases calcium and phosphate resorption (calcitriol). Increases bone formation (24-hydroxy-calcidiol).	Increases calcium and phosphate resorption (high doses). Possibly increases bone formation (low doses).	Little initial effect. Long term decrease in rates of bone resorption and formation.
Kidney	Decreases excretion of calcium and phosphate (calcidiol and calcitriol).	Decreases calcium excretion but increases phosphate excretion.	Increases calcium and phosphate excretion.
Blood Plasma	Overall increase in calcium and phosphate levels.	Overall increase in calcium level but decrease in phosphate level.	Overall decrease in calcium and Phosphate levels

Table 60.5. Vitamin D compendium

FOOD GROUP	VITAMIN D LEVEL
Milk and products	Very low
Eggs	Medium
Meat and fish	Very variable
Fats and oils	Very variable
Grain and products	Nil
Nuts and pulses	Nil
Root vegetables	Nil
Leaf vegetables	Nil
Fruit	Nil
Sweets	Nil

61

Are There Other Vitamins?

It can be seen from the historical notes in the preceding chapters on the vitamins that most of the discoveries regarding the vitamins occurred in the first half of the last century. Also, it can be seen from the multitude of alternative names associated with the vitamins (Table 61.1) that considerable confusion must have arisen over the years. Therefore, it is convenient to repeat that there are only fourteen vitamins (see Tables 46.1 and 46.2) that are considered to be essential for human nutrition. Although, in the general literature, a few other vitamin-like nutrients are sometimes considered in this category.

During the early years, a large number of different factors were under investigation. Many of these were also assigned letters and numbers as was the custom at the time. On further purification, it was shown that several of these differently named substances were in fact identical, and some of the alternative names had to be dropped. Also, further study showed that not all of these factors were true vitamins (at least as far as human nutrition was concerned). Thus, there arose various gaps in both the numbering and the lettering systems.

Since the original discoveries, it has been found that most vitamins have companions of closely related structure (vitamers) which have similar biological properties. Such related substances are best referred to using generic descriptors. Each descriptor is simply a letter or a word that embraces all such substances of a given biological activity and similar structure.

Thus, while vitamin A was originally believed to be a single substance, the term is now used to include many substances such as alcohols, aldehydes and acids that are derivatives of retinol and possess antixerophthalmic activity. Indeed, approximately 50 carotenoids are now known to possess such activity in varying degrees. In addition, the term niacin is now a generic descriptor for nicotinic acid and all its derivatives with antipellagric activity. And, the term folate is a generic descriptor for folic acid and all its derivatives with antianaemic activity.

The accompanying Table 61.1 lists various designations both old and new, and identifies some of their various usages.

Table 61.1.i. Identity of vitamin designations (mostly obsolete)

LABEL	IDENTITY
A	A generic descriptor for all β–ionone derivatives (except provitamin A), with antixerophthalmic activity.
A_1	Retinol-1 or retinol$_1$.
A_2	Retinol-2 or retinol$_2$.
B	Represents the group of all B vitamins and several related compounds which are not true vitamins for humans.
B_1	Thiamin.
B_2	Riboflavin. Occasionally used in the past to represent all the vitamins except thiamin or more specifically a group consisting of niacin, riboflavin, pantothenic acid, biotin and choline.
B_3	Together with niacin, best used as a generic descriptor for all compounds exhibiting qualitatively the biological activity of nicotinic acid. Occasionally used in the past to represent pantothenic acid.
B_4	A mixture consisting of some activity that prevents muscular weakness in rats or chickens. Originally thought to be adenine. Either a mixture of glycine, arginine and cysteine or a mixture of riboflavin and pyridoxine. Also, used for thiamin or biotin.
B_5	A growth stimulator in pigeons. Probably niacin. Also, best used for pantothenic acid.
B_6	A generic descriptor for all derivatives of 2methylpyridine with the activity of pyridoxine.
B_7	Used for some unspecified activity that prevents digestive disturbances in pigeons. Also, has been used for nicotinic acid. Probably best used as a generic descriptor for all compounds exhibiting qualitatively the biological activity of D-biotin.
B_8	Adenylic acid, a growth factor for certain bacteria. Also, used for inositol.

Table 61.1.ii.

LABEL	IDENTITY
B_9	Used to designate some factor for bacteria. Probably best used as a generic descriptor for all compounds exhibiting qualitatively the biological activity of folate.
B_{10}	Used for some activity that promotes feathering in chickens, probably folate and vitamin B_{12}. Once used for pteroylmonoglutamic acid. Also, used for *para*-aminobenzoic acid (PABA).
B_{11}	Probably identical to B_{10}. Sometimes used for salicylic acid or pteryl-hepta-glutamic acid.
B_{12}	A generic descriptor for cobalamin and all its derivatives with antipernicious anaemia activity. In the past, various derivatives have been given numbers such as 12a for aquocobalamin, 12b for hydrocobalamin, and 12c for nitrocobalamin. Other numbers used included 12r, 12s, 12III, and V_{1a}. Such designations are no longer in use.
B_{13}	An unconfirmed factor, probably orotic acid.
B_{14}	A substance found in human urine that promotes cell growth in the bone marrow, probably vitamin B_{12} or one of its derivatives.
B_{15}	Pangamic acid.
B_{16}	Never assigned.
B_{17}	Laetrile (amygdalin), a factor claimed to inhibit the growth of cancer cells or kill them.
B_c	Folate.
B_p	An activity that prevents perosis in chickens probably choline and manganese.
B_t	An activity that promotes growth in insects and mealworms, probably carnitine. Sometimes written as BT.

Table 61.1.iii.

LABEL	IDENTITY
B_W	Probably biotin.
B_X	*para*-Aminobenzoic acid, or occasionally pantothenic acid.
C	A generic descriptor for ascorbic acid and related compounds with antiscorbutic activity.
C_2	Some unknown activity claimed to prevent pneumonia. Also, used for mixture of substances called bioflavonoids found in association with vitamin C.
D	A generic descriptor for all secosteroid derivatives with antirachitic activity.
D_1	A mixture of vitamin D_2 and lumisterol. No longer in use.
D_2	Ergocalciferol, and activated derivatives.
D_3	Cholecalciferol, and activated derivatives.
E	A generic descriptor for all tocopherol and tocotrienol derivatives with α–tocopherol activity.
E_1	α–Tocopherol.
E_2	β–Tocopherol.
E_3	γ–Tocopherol. These designations are not in general use.
F	A mixture of essential fatty acids, particularly linoleic acid, α–linolenic acid and arachidonic acid.
Factor S	Salicylic acid.
Factor X	Vitamin E
Folacin	An obsolete term for folic acid or any of its derivatives that has the biological activity of tetrahydrofolic acid.
G	Riboflavin.
H	Biotin. Also, used for *para*-aminobenzoic acid.
H_3	Procaine, not a vitamin. Sometimes called GH_3 or gerovital.

Table 61.1.iv.

LABEL	IDENTITY
I	Same as B_7.
J	Identical to the pneumonia preventative factor called C_2.
K	A generic descriptor for all derivatives of menadione with antihaemorrhagic activity (including menadione itself).
K_1	Phylloquinone. Often referred to simply as K.
K_2	Various menaquinones
K_3	Menadione, a water soluble synthetic form of vitamin K.
K_4	The di-hydroxy derivative of menadione.
K_5	Synkamin or 2-methyl-4-amino-1-naphthol.
L_1	Liver filtrate, probably anthranilic acid (an isomer of *para*-aminobenzoic acid).
L_2	Yeast filtrate, probably adenosine. L_1 and L_2 are believed to be lactation factors for rats but are not significant in humans.
M	Some activity that prevents blood disorders including anaemia in monkeys, probably folate.
N	Unknown extract of brain or stomach once believed to inhibit cancer.
NE	Niacin Equivalent. The term includes the contribution of nicotinic acid, nicotinamide and tryptophan to the total niacin activity.
P	Bioflavonoids.
PP	Nicotinic acid.
R	Some activity that promotes bacterial growth, probably folate.

Table 61.1.v.

LABEL	IDENTITY
RE	Retinol Equivalent. The term (used up to 2001) includes the contribution of β-carotene and other provitamins to the total vitamin A activity. However, the contribution factors were based on inaccurate data.
RAE	Retinol Activity Equivalent. The term (used since 2001) includes the contribution of β-carotene and other provitamins to the total vitamin A activity.
S	Some activity that promotes the growth of certain bacteria, probably related to the peptide streptogenin which contains cysteine and leucine.
T	Unspecified group of substances originally isolated from termites (called termitin) and other insects (insectine), yeasts and moulds (penicin, a precursor of penicillin), and sesame seeds (sesame seed factor), that promotes protein assimilation in the rat. Probably a mixture of nucleic acid derivatives, folate and vitamin B_{12}. Also, called Goetsch's factor.
THFA	Tetrahydrofolic acid
TE	Tocopherol Equivalent. The term includes the contribution of all tocols and tocotrienols to the total vitamin E activity.
U	Cabbage extract that cures ulcers, probably vitamin B_6 and folate. Also, contains methionine derivatives.
V	Some activity that promotes growth in bacteria, probably the cofactor NAD (nicotinamide adenine dinucleotide).
Vitamin R	Pteroylmonoglutamic acid.
X	Frequently used over the years to represent any new factor.

62

Some Links Between the Nutrients

The major vitamins were all discovered in the period 1926 to 1948. However, it is only since 1948 that the analysis of many trace elements became accurate enough to enable their evaluation as essential nutrients. Most vitamins and all minerals and trace elements are obtained from the food we eat. Minerals and trace elements ultimately derive from the soil or the sea which supports plants and animals during growth. Vitamins derive primarily from plant foods or from the gut bacteria. Also, they occur in animals which eat other animals. In a few cases, animals can synthesise certain vitamins themselves. Even though each essential mineral and vitamin is uniquely important in its own right, special links or relationships often exist between them. Some aspects of these relationships will be considered in this chapter.

Blood

One area where a number of minerals and vitamins work together is in the maintenance of the correct composition of the blood, notably with regard to the formation of the red blood cell (or erythrocyte). These cells are essential for oxygen transport and deficiencies of the red blood cells are termed anaemias. At its simplest, anaemia may be defined as a reduction in the total number of red blood cells. Anaemia may also be considered as an insufficiency in the function of the red blood cells. Because the number, the size, and the haemoglobin content, of red blood cells can vary under different conditions to produce anaemia, the total mass of the circulating red blood cells is often considered to be the most useful index of assessment. In practice, however, the haemoglobin content of the blood gives a simple measure of the ability of the cells to carry out their respiratory function. If the total haemoglobin content per litre of blood lies below the normal range, then anaemia can be said to be present. Red cells have an average lifespan of 120 to 130 days, which means that around 1 percent of the red blood cell must be replaced every day to prevent anaemia from developing. Consequently, about 8 to 10 grams of haemoglobin must be synthesised per day to maintain this turnover, and to ensure that each red cell can efficiently carry out its function. Red blood cells are formed in the bone marrow from precursor cells.

Anaemia may be caused by impaired production of red blood cells, increased breakdown of red blood cells (haemolysis), or directly by blood loss. Anaemias may be genetic or acquired. The acquired anaemias are the main ones of interest in nutrition. Production of red blood cells may be decreased due to a deficiency of the hormone called erythropoietin which stimulates red cell differentiation in the bone marrow. Haemolytic anaemias may be caused by fevers or infections, or by disturbances in the levels of certain enzymes. Interestingly, the lack of almost any essential nutrient can lead to anaemia in the long term. However, certain key nutrients are associated more directly with different types of anaemia. Of these, only a few need to be considered here. Protein deficiency states such as protein-energy malnutrition, or even the lack of certain individual essential amino acids, leads to anaemia in humans.

Of the minerals, iron is obviously the most essential in preventing anaemia, but copper and other trace elements are also essential for proper utilization of iron in the body. Regarding iron itself, it is not often realised that, commonly, half of the total iron loss in young women is due to blood loss during menstruation (which averages about 35 ml of blood per month). Hence, the marked difference in the recommended daily intakes for men and women in this age group. Pregnancy also markedly increases the need for iron.

Of the vitamins, vitamin B_{12} is the most important in preventing pernicious anaemia. The underlying cause of pernicious anaemia is not yet fully understood. It is not directly due to a lack of vitamin B_{12} itself in the diet, but to a factor in the gastric juice which is essential for the absorption of the vitamin. The lack of other vitamins may also result in different types of anaemia. Folate deficiency is associated with anaemia, particularly in young children. This is due to a deficiency in haemoglobin synthesis due to diminished synthesis of nucleic acids in the young red blood cell and this leads to macrocytic or megaloblastic anaemia. Vitamin B_6 deficiency may lead to a form of microcytic anaemia in certain animals but this is rare in humans. Vitamin C is important for the absorption of iron, because it helps convert iron to the more easily absorbed ferrous form. Vitamin E has a role to play in preventing anaemia in infants. It should be clear from the above summary that a well-balanced diet is the best defence against anaemia, although for some women iron supplementation may also be required.

Vitamins and Minerals

Perhaps the best-known relationship between vitamins and minerals is the relationship between vitamin D and calcium. This relationship is compounded further by the relationship between calcium and phosphate which, at its simplest, may be summarised by the rule-of-thumb, 'calcium times phosphate is a constant'. This means that if calcium concentration increases in a fluid, then the phosphate concentration decreases proportionally, and *vice versa*. This relationship has been questioned in recent years and may not hold true in all fluids (in a strictly mathematical sense). Nevertheless, as a rule-of-thumb, it is a useful concept to work with in general nutrition.

More recently, the special relationship between vitamin E and selenium has been elucidated. Also, there is a relationship where vitamin C can enhance the absorption of iron by converting ferric to ferrous iron. And, there appears to be a relationship between vitamin A and zinc, where zinc promotes the release of vitamin A from the liver stores to ensure good night vision. Finally, it could be argued that the strongest possible relationship exists for vitamin B_{12} and cobalt, where the cobalt serves as an intrinsic component of the vitamin structure. Indeed, cobalt itself has no known function in the human body outside this unique structural role. But vitamin B_{12} cannot function on its own in the formation of normal red blood cells. In this function, at least, it requires the close cooperation of folate.

Electrolytes

Relationships may be general or highly specific. For example, there are general relationships between several of the minerals. Many of the minerals act as electrolytes in the body. Electrolytes are charged particles called ions which carry either positive or negative charges. The total number of positive charges in any given solution equals the total number of negative charges. Also, irrespective of whether a particle has a charge or not, the total number of particles inside the cell must equal the total number of particles outside the cell in order to maintain osmotic balance and prevent too much water either entering or leaving the cell. In this regard, it does not matter what the nature of the particles are, as long as their grand totals are equal. In fact, for any given mineral, there will be an uneven distribution across the cell membrane. Some minerals have a naturally greater concentration inside the cell in the intracellular fluid. Whereas, other minerals have a naturally greater concentration outside the cell in the extracellular fluid (which has essentially the same composition as blood plasma). Table 46.1 illustrates the distribution of several electrolytes across a typical cell membrane in the human body.

The individual electrolytes are linked, insofar as the total charge needs to be neutral, and the total concentration of particles on both sides of a membrane needs to be the same. Given this constraint, there is still considerable flexibility. With regard to the figures given in Table 62.1, these are all expressed in terms of milligrams per litre. However, for any given substance, the actual number of particles per milligram depends on the size of the particle, or strictly its molar mass. That is one reason why the totals on both sides do not necessarily add up to give the same total value. Another reason is that there are many other chemical substances, particularly organic substances, and especially proteins, which contribute to the final distribution. Nevertheless, Table 62.1 clearly shows the uneven distribution of many substances in the body. A disturbance in the concentration of any one of these minerals at any point, therefore, tends to cause a change in several electrolytes at the same time.

Table 62.1. Chief electrolyte content of body fluids (all values in milligrams per litre)

ELECTROLYTE	SYMBOL	CELL WATER (Intracellular fluid)	BLOOD PLASMA (Extracellular fluid)
Potassium	K^+	5,800	200
Sodium	Na^+	250	3,400
Chloride	Cl^-	500	4,200
Phosphate	P_i	5,800	200
Bicarbonate	HCO_3^-	600	1,700
Calcium	Ca_2^{2+}	trace	100
Magnesium	Mg_2^{2+}	500	50
Sulphate	SO_4^{2-}	1,000	100

Phosphate is expressed as total inorganic phosphate (P_i) and includes the two forms $H_2PO_4^-$ and HPO_4^{2-}.

Bicarbonate is formed from water and carbon dioxide by the following reactions in the body: $H_2O + CO_2 = H_2CO_3 = H^+ + HCO_3^-$.

63

Some Nonvitamins
Bioflavonoids, L-Carnitine, Phospholipid Factors, para-Aminobenzoic Acid, Taurine, Nucleic Acid Factors, Lipoic Acid, Pangamic Acid and Laetrile.

There are only fourteen recognised vitamins as far as human nutrition is concerned. Therefore, it follows logically that all other nutrients are not vitamins. However, several substances which are usually associated with the vitamins in nature also have biological effects. These effects can be vitamin-like and indeed for some species, but not for humans, these substances actually are vitamins. In this book, we refer to such substances as nonvitamins. Other authors have termed them substances without vitamin status, vitaminoids, or even inaccurately as vitamins.

There are two main reasons why such substances are termed nonvitamins rather than vitamins. One reason may be the fact that the substance is not nutritionally essential for life even though it may have certain therapeutic effects. Such substances include the bioflavonoid, and two dubious ones, pangamic acid and laetrile. Another reason why a substance may be termed a nonvitamin is the fact that it may be synthesised in the body (or in the gut) at a rate sufficient to fulfil all the needs of the body. The other nonvitamins considered in this chapter fall into this class, but these can also have certain therapeutic effects associated with them. To further distinguish between nonvitamins and other pharmacological substances the term is confined to natural substances with so-called vitamin-like properties and which are generally found in association with the vitamins in nature. It is possible that some of the nonvitamins may verge on becoming contingent in certain circumstances.

Now because all the substances discussed in this chapter are nonvitamins, there is strictly no daily requirement for any of them, consequently there should be no deficiency symptoms associated with the lack of them in the diet, at least in normal healthy individuals. Some of the nonvitamins were listed previously in Table 46.3. These will now be considered.

Bioflavonoids

Around 1936 Szent-Györgyi and others found that crude extracts of vitamin C contained another factor called citrin, vitamin P or vitamin C_2, that co-operated with the biological effects of pure vitamin C. Citrin was later shown to be a mixture of substances called flavonoids. These have been given a variety of names such as vitamin J, anti-pneumonia factor, citrus fruit factor, paprika factor, permeability factor, and so on. In 1950, it was recognised that these substances, although of therapeutic interest, were not essential and the general term bioflavonoids was adopted.

There are over 4,000 flavonoids found in plants, some of them are free and others are combined with glucose (glucosides). Flavonoids are polyphenolic compounds that occur ubiquitously in plants. They generally contain a common chemical structure called 2-phenyl-1,4-benzopyrone which consists of three aromatic rings. Often these compounds are brightly coloured. Ivory, yellow, red, purple, blue or violet are the most common colours which function as plant pigments. The colours depend on the number of hydroxyl (–OH), and methyl (–CH$_3$) groups attached to the basic structure. The bioflavonoids consist of flavonones. flavones, flavonols and a further nine chemical types.

The individual compounds most frequently mentioned include the following: quercetin, hesperidin, rutin, naringin, eriodictyol, nobiletin. heptamethoxy flavone, myricetin, kaempferol, tangeritin, sinensetin and phlorhizin. With a few exceptions, these need not be considered separately. Hesperidin is a flavone glycoside which constitutes 8 percent of the dry weight of orange peel. Many of the bioflavonoids have functions similar to hesperidin. Rutin is the most common flavonol, and is a yellow glycoside (rhamnoglucose) derivative of quercetin found in buckwheat. Naringin is another similar derivative. Phlorhizin is a dihydroxychalcone found in root bark. It is poisonous and blocks glucose retention by the kidneys.

Bioflavonoids aid the assimilation and function of vitamin C. Bioflavonoids in general reduce the fragility and permeability of tiny blood vessels called capillaries. One theory is that the bioflavonoids may act as antioxidants and thus spare vitamin C which is the essential vitamin maintaining capillary integrity. Quercetin and related compounds may inhibit the enzyme *O*-methyltransferase which is involved in the metabolism of adrenaline and related hormones. Quercetin may also inhibit the enzyme aldose reductase which has been claimed to be involved in cataract formation in certain diabetic patients. Compounds with this type of action are the hydroxylated bioflavonoids such as quercetin, myricetin and kaempferol. The bioflavonoids have been found beneficial for certain menstrual problems and for varicose veins, bruising, bleeding and haemorrhoids. The anti-inflammatory action of several of the bioflavonoids may be beneficial in treating certain forms of rheumatism, arthritis and related problems. Bioflavonoids have also been tested as protective agents against certain forms of radiation. Some methoxylated bioflavonoids may prevent stickiness of the blood platelets. Others possess anti-infective properties and it has been claimed may assist vitamin C in warding off colds. Nobiletin itself has an anti-inflammatory action and, like tangeretin, may also act as a detoxifying agent. Rutin has a specific antihypertensive action and has been used to control mildly high blood pressure. Rutin may also be beneficial in treating arteriosclerosis.

It has been estimated that the typical average intake of bioflavonoids is around 200 mg per day. Most countries have not set a daily allowance, although two Eastern Bloc countries recommend some 16 - 20 mg, as a minimum daily intake. This amount is certainly greatly exceeded in most diets. The best sources are fruits, especially citrus fruits (skins, peels and the central core or pith), apricots, blackberries, black currants, cherries, grapes, plumbs and rose hips. Good vegetable sources include peppers, tomatoes, red onions and broccoli. Buckwheat is the best source of rutin.

Bioflavonoids are non-toxic. For example, several grams of hesperidin per day for prolonged periods had no adverse effects on humans. Rutin is also available as a supplement. Because of its unique action in lowering blood pressure, care should be taken if using this form of flavonol. Several flavonoids are poisonous such as phlorhizin, but these are not taken as nutrients in the diet. Excessive amounts of bioflavonoids are excreted rapidly in the urine. There are no deficiency symptoms associated with the bioflavonoids.

L-Carnitine

Tenebrio molitor is a close member of the vitamin B group. It is a polar water-soluble compound with the chemical name, γ–trimethylamino–β–hydroxybutyric acid. The D-isomer is inactive. Carnitine can be synthesised slowly in the body in the presence of vitamin C and is found in all animal tissues particularly in muscle and in liver. It was first isolated from meat extracts in Russia in 1905. The mealworm, *Tenebrio molitor*, requires carnitine as a vitamin, hence the name vitamin B_t. Its structure was established in 1952. In adult humans, the substance is not required because it can be synthesised. However, it has been reported recently that a rare muscle disorder can be treated by administering carnitine at a level of 40 mg per day. Hence, it may become a conditionally essential dietary requirement in certain circumstances. Also in infants, it has been suggested that L-carnitine may be contingent in certain cases.

L-Carnitine is essential for the transport of lipid in the cell. It is located on the mitochondrial membrane and controls the rate of transport of fatty acids across the membrane and also the permeability of the membrane. In the absence of carnitine, there is a buildup of fat in the form of triacylglycerols in the cell. Carnitine may therefore act as a lipid mobiliser. There is no evidence the carnitine in the diet is toxic.

Phospholipid Factors
Choline and *myo*-Inositol

Popularly called lecithin, there are in fact several different types of phospholipid, which are characterised by the moiety attached to the phosphate part of the parent compound called phosphatidic acid. If this moiety is choline, then the compound is called phosphatidylcholine or lecithin proper. If the moiety is *myo*-inositol, then the compound is called phosphatidylinositol or lipositol. Sometimes other entities such as the amino acid serine or ethanolamine may be attached to the phosphate. Phosphatidic acid itself consists of four units; a central glycerol unit (consisting of a three-carbon unit), two fatty acids and a phosphate group. Approximately equivalent amounts of choline and inositol are available in the average diet, mainly as phospholipid components although they also occur in other forms. When free, both choline and inositol are water-soluble and are associated with the B-group vitamins.

Choline

Choline is widely distributed in plants and animals. In the past, choline has been referred to as amantine, bilineurine, gossypine, vidine, chicken antiperosis factor and even vitamin B_p. It occurs in the phospholipid lecithin and also in the nerve transmitter acetylcholine which was first synthesised in 1867. The role of acetylcholine in the nervous system was not however fully realised until about 1921. Free choline occurs as a trimethylammonium salt. Choline is involved primarily with the utilization of lipids and cholesterol in the body. It prevents the accumulation of fat in the liver by promoting its transport. Hence the designation lipid mobiliser, fat-fighter or anti-fat agent. Choline together with the amino acid methionine is involved in transfer of methyl ($-CH_3$) groups by a process called transmethylation. Choline is essential for maintaining the nerve cell coverings. These so-called myelin sheaths cover the long processes of the nerve cells called axons, and thus aid in the transmission of nervous impulses. Choline may also help to prevent the formation of gallstones. Together with folate, vitamin B_{12} and methionine, choline helps resist infection. Choline may strengthen the walls of capillary vessels, and has been used therapeutically to improve blood flow to the eyes. Choline may relieve insomnia in certain individuals, and also palpitations, dizziness and ear noises. The best sources of choline include liver, egg yolks, grains, pulses and nuts, yeast and lecithin itself. There is no toxicity associated with choline in the diet. Massive doses however may deplete vitamin B_6 if prolonged.

A deficiency of choline cannot be produced in the presence of adequate protein in the diet. In experimental animals, a deficiency results in impaired lipid transport and mobilisation, resulting in fatty livers. Prolonged deficiency may also cause ulcers. In animals, there results kidney damage, anaemia and lowered blood pressure, but these effects have not been observed in humans. In certain cases, deficiency has been implicated with high blood pressure and atherosclerosis. In 1998, choline was classified as an essential nutrient and is usually grouped within the B-group vitamins.

myo-Inositol

Inositol was first isolated from muscle in 1850, by Scherrer. There are nine isomers of inositol, but only the form called *myo*-inositol is biologically active. *myo*-Inositol is a water-soluble substance sometimes called *i*-inositol, bios I, inosite, *meso*-inositol, cyclohexitol, hexahydrocyclohexane or even its full chemical name *cis*-1,2,3,5-*trans*-4,6-cyclohexanehexol. Inositol is a close relative of the carbohydrate glucose. In plants, particularly grains, inositol may occur as the hexaphosphate called phytic acid, or as a mixed calcium and magnesium salt of phytic acid called phytin. Excess of phytic acid may therefore cause a lack of available calcium resulting in rickets, if prolonged. Phytic acid may also interfere with the absorption of magnesium, iron and zinc. Other forms of inositol include the mono-, di- and tri-, phosphoric esters which are often linked to other carbohydrates. Rich sources of inositol are seeds, grains, pulses and nuts, yeast and certain fruits. In animal tissues, it occurs as a component of phospholipids. *myo*-Inositol is well digested and absorbed from the gut, and it may be synthesised slowly in the body. Large quantities are found in liver, heart and skeletal muscle. Lecithin itself is an excellent source.

A major function of inositol relates to its role as a phospholipid component of all cell membranes. It is therefore involved in maintaining the permeability of membranes, assisting in hormone binding to the cell surface, and in enabling nerve impulses to be properly transmitted. *myo*-Inositol may be converted to glucose and *vice versa*. Large doses may alleviate the ketosis caused by the absence of carbohydrates. *myo*-Inositol, like choline, promotes the mobilization of lipids especially from the liver. It may also help to lower blood cholesterol levels, if administered a rate of 2 grams per day for several weeks. Inositol may improve the appearance of the hair.

It has been estimated that some 85 mg *myo*-inositol per 1,000 kJ (360 mg per 1,000 kcal), is obtained from the average diet. The average intake per day could therefore be around 1,000 mg. Inositol is non-toxic. Although experimental doses around 30 grams per day caused diarrhoea in some humans. Under normal circumstances a deficiency never occurs in humans, although excessive amounts of coffee tend to deplete inositol levels. Inositol acts as a vitamin in several animal species. In certain laboratory animals, a dietary deficiency resulted in a loss of hair, hence the older designations mouse anti-alopecia factor and rat anti-spectacle eye factor. Other animals require it as a store of energy in muscle, notably the shark. Lipid disorders may occur in animals deprived of *myo*-inositol. These disorders relate to lack of mobilization of lipid especially in the liver. Therapeutic doses of inositol may be beneficial for certain patients with liver problems.

para-Aminobenzoic Acid

para-Aminobenzoic acid, alternatively termed PABA, *para*-aminobenzoate or 4-aminobenzoic acid, is a component of folic acid. For this reason, it has been termed a vitamin within a vitamin. Other terms used to describe it include rat anti-gray-hair factor, cosmetic factor, achromotrichia factor, vitamin B_x, bacterial vitamin

H (or H'), and the anticanitic vitamin.

Some organisms require PABA for growth but it is not itself required in human nutrition although it must be supplied in the form of folate which is essential. Some organisms, but not humans, are able to synthesise folate from PABA. PABA is a water-soluble compound found in association with the B-group vitamins in nature.

PABA may be beneficial in promoting the growth of bacteria in the gut. The growth inhibiting effects of sulfanilamide (sulfa drugs) on certain bacteria is counteracted by PABA. In certain skin conditions where blanching of the skin occurs, high doses of PABA helps to restore the normal pigmentation. Another therapeutic use of PABA is as a sun screening agent to prevent sunburn. Sometimes, oral preparations are used but topical lotions are preferable. PABA also sooths the pain of burns.

Natural sources of PABA include liver, eggs, yeast and whole grains. PABA is relatively nontoxic. Doses up to several grams per day may be administered for short periods. High doses, however, may cause nausea and irritation of the skin, and prolonged intakes may cause liver and kidney damage. One sign of deficiency in certain animals is the premature greying of hair. It is sometimes claimed that PABA, especially in combination with folate and pantothenic acid, has the effect of restoring colour to grey hair in humans but this is uncertain. A prolonged deficiency may result in digestive upsets.

Taurine

The chemical name for taurine is β–aminoethanesulfonic acid. Taurine can be synthesised from cysteine or methionine in the liver. Therefore, it is not considered nutritionally essential for humans except perhaps in rare circumstances. For example, infants fed on taurine-deficient formula milk have lower plasma levels of taurine than infants fed on breast milk. Low levels of zinc tend to increase the levels of taurine circulating in blood plasma but decrease the levels in the brain. Because taurine is one of the inhibitory neurotransmitters, low levels may predispose to epilepsy. Restriction of sulphur-containing amino acids in the diet may also reduce the levels of taurine. The female hormone estradiol depresses the formation of taurine.

Taurine is essential for the formation of one type of bile salt, namely conjugated taurocholic acid. This salt is a particularly good biological detergent which helps to maintain the solubility of cholesterol in bile. High concentrations of taurine are also found in blood platelets. Taurine spares potassium and calcium loss from heart muscle. Taurine also influences blood glucose levels.

In animal studies, large oral doses of taurine have been shown to stimulate the production of growth hormone. The synthesis of taurine is limited in cats. Deficiency in cats can result in eye problems, spontaneous abortions, poor growth rate in kittens, heart disease and a lowered immunity to infections.

Nucleic Acid Factors
Adenine, Adenylic Acid and Orotic Acid

Adenine, adenylic acid and orotic acid have all at one time been claimed to be vitamins. It is now known that these compounds can be synthesised in the body, although they may be required as vitamins for the growth of certain bacteria.

Adenine itself is one of the two purines found in nucleic acids. When combined with ribose-5-phosphate it produces the compound called adenylic acid, which is one of the nucleotides. Adenylic acid is also called adenosine monophosphate (or AMP for short). Other purine and pyrimidine bases give rise to other such nucleotides which are essential as coenzymes, and for the synthesis of DNA and RNA.

Orotic acid, which has been called whey factor, milk factor, animal galactose factor, factor B_{13} and even vitamin B_{13} (incorrectly), is a metabolic precursor of the pyrimidines. Three pyrimidines occur in nucleic acids and all of these can be synthesised in the body in normal individuals. Excessive intake of purines may contribute to gout in certain individuals. A deficiency of nucleic acid factors does not occur in normal individuals.

Lipoic Acid

Lipoic acid, also called α-lipoic acid, lipoate or 6-thioctic acid, is found in muscle. It is required as a vitamin for the protozoan called *Tetrahymena geleii*, and several other organisms. It was first isolated in 1951 by Reed, *et al*. Humans can synthesise lipoic acid in extremely small amounts necessary for metabolism of certain central metabolic intermediates. Lipoic acid, also called 1,2-dithiolane-3-valeric acid, is a disulfide derivative of octanoic acid. It is a unique fat-soluble substance not related to any of the other vitamins or nonvitamins. Like biotin, it may be linked to enzymes by lysine residues thus acting as a coenzyme for acyl transfer reactions.

Together with several ether coenzymes including thiamin pyrophosphate, coenzyme A, nicotinamide adeninedinucleotide, and flavin adeninedinucleotide, it is involved in the decarboxylation of keto acid intermediates of metabolism. For example, pyruvate decarboxylase is a multienzyme system involving these coenzymes in a highly organised molecular complex. It is interesting that this one reaction involving the removal of a carboxyl group (–COOH) from keto acids such as pyruvate and the liberation of free carbon dioxide (CO_2), requires coenzymes containing derivatives of lipoic acid, thiamin, niacin, riboflavin and pantothenic acid. During these reactions, lipoic acid is reversibly oxidised and reduced.

Another function of lipoic acid may be the inactivation of free cyanide ions which react rapidly with the cyclic disulfide group in the acid's ring structure. Lipoic acid only occurs in minute amounts and so there are no reports of toxicity or deficiency symptoms.

Pangamic Acid

Pangamic acid was first discovered in 1951 by Krebs and Krebs, is a water-soluble ester of D-gluconic and dimethylaminoacetic acids (dimethylglycine). Synthetic forms are also water-soluble substances of uncertain composition, but probably consists of either N,N-diisopropylamine dichloroacetate or N-diisopropylglycine glucuronate or a mixture of dimethylglycine and sorbitol, which has the effect of decreasing blood pressure and temperature in certain laboratory animals. Pangamic acid is widely distributed in nature, and occurs in association with other members of the B-group vitamins. It has been called pangamate, factor B_{15} and even vitamin B_{15} (incorrectly). It occurs in apricot kernels, whole grains including brown rice, certain seeds, yeast and liver.

Pangamic acid promotes cellular respiration and glucose oxidation. It promotes the availability of oxygen to many tissues especially muscle and the heart. It may therefore have some therapeutic use in oxygen deficiency diseases such as asthma and angina. It is claimed that pangamic acid can relieve the feeling of tiredness, protect the liver from cirrhosis and reduce the craving for alcohol in certain chronic alcoholic patients. Pangamic acid may act as a lipotropic agent and may be of benefit in atherosclerosis. Pangamic acid, being a methyl ($-CH_3$) donor may also function as a detoxifying agent. Like vitamins C and E, pangamic acid may act as an antioxidant. Pangamic acid stimulates the elevation of anti-stress hormones in the blood. And it has been claimed may help to prevent certain cancers. Research on this substance is continuing in the Russia.

Pangamic acid is generally nontoxic. Extremely high doses may be toxic, particularly of the dichloro- form, which causes flushing of the skin. There are no deficiency symptoms associated with pangamic acid in humans.

Laetrile

Laetrile, whose full chemical name is laevo-mandelonitrile-β–glucuronoside, is also known as amygdalin, bitter almond factor, apricot kernel factor, factor B_{17} and even vitamin B_{17} (incorrectly).

Amygdalin which is the natural form of laetrile is found in apricot kernels and many other nuts and seeds, is a water-soluble substance and has been used in cancer therapy for over 140 years, with spurious results. Laetrile is a semisynthetic form derived from amygdalin and has a similar structure. Laetrile belongs to group of substances called nitrilosides which contain cyanide. This cyanide is organically bound and is considered harmless. It has been estimated that the daily intake of amygdalin and other nitrilosides amounts to several milligrams. Apart from fruit kernels and seeds, smaller amounts are found in sweet potatoes, corn millet, and certain pulses and nuts. Certain grasses and foliage contain significant amounts of nitrilosides and the meat of animals that graze on these crops may also contain increased amounts of the substance.

Normal body cells only liberate the poisonous cyanide from the organic nitrilosides extremely slowly. However, the rationale behind their use as anticancer agents is theoretically interesting. It can be shown that certain cancer cells contain high concentrations of enzyme called β–glucosidase that breaks down laetrile and releases cyanide. This cyanide in turn is supposed to kill off the cells which release it but should not affect normal body cells. In practice, however, it is found that the cyanide leaks out of the cancer cells and may buildup in the body causing serious toxicity and even death. Unfortunately, for the treatment to work (assuming that it does work at all) very large doses of laetrile must be given and serious complications cannot be avoided.

Even normal cells can release small amounts of cyanide from the nitrilosides. This is where a second enzyme comes into play. The enzyme, oddly called rhodanese, neutralises free cyanide. This enzyme occurs in normal cells but is deficient in cancer cells. In theory, this is another advantage. However, so much laetrile must be used that the enzyme is overwhelmed and cyanide levels buildup in the body. But in theory the cancer cells are more susceptible to cyanide poisoning than normal cells. It is one thing to show an effect on a few cells in a test tube. It is quite another to produce the same effect in the whole body.

Nitrilosides are not toxic in low doses. Mild toxic effects include headaches, nausea and low blood pressure. An average apricot kernel contains about 5 mg (although some may contain up to 30 mg) amygdalin. The kernels are usually crushed and made into a slurry. Not more that 15 kernels should be taken throughout a day. More than one gram should never be taken at any one time. It may be more pleasant to eat a few bitter almonds from time to time. No deficiency symptoms of amygdalin have been reported. Following studies on the eating habits of Eskimos and Hunzakuts, it has been suggested a prolonged deficiency of nitrilosides in the diet may predispose to certain types of malignancy. Laetrile has been discredited by the US Food and Drug Administration.

64

Trace Poisons

In various chapters in this book the point was made that a mixed and varied diet was more appropriate than strictly limited regimes. One reason for this, taking amino acids for example, is that the effective quality of protein in a diet can be improved by mixing. Another is the fact that different foods have different combinations and amounts of vitamins and minerals. Yet another good reason for variety is the presence of certain trace poisons even in the most naturally grown foods. And food that is not grown naturally, such as most of the meat, fruit and vegetables on sale today, contains some additional contaminants that can affect health. In many respects, the purist has Hobson's choice of choosing between either animal produce containing traces of antibiotics and hormones or vegetable produce containing traces of pesticide residues and natural poisons, even if these are at absolutely minimal levels. In recent years, food processors have been forced to label the contents of their products many of which contain artificial additives (some of which may have adverse effects in susceptible individuals). Thankfully, the food industry is more aware than ever of the importance of limiting or eliminating all sources of unnecessary contamination and adulteration.

Observing the rules of hygiene and the proper storing and cooking of food reduces the risk of infections, particularly these of bacterial origin. These rules cannot however remove traces of toxins, heavy metals, radioactivity, and so on, that are occasionally present in extremely low concentrations. But there is absolutely no need for alarm because the golden rules of moderation and variety can ensure the maximum protection of health, even in less than ideal circumstances. High intakes of certain non-nutrients, such as cholesterol, are inadvisable. Too much of any nutrient can represent a potential long-term risk. Plant foods themselves are the chief source of actual organic poisons that can represent another potential risk if overeaten. Table 63.1 lists a number of poisons which occur naturally in vegetable and some animal foods. The list may surprise some, but it is just as bad to be scare-mongered into avoiding nutritious foodstuffs as it is to be selectively over-indulgent in eating any of them. Most of us regularly eat many of the foods listed in the table without any misadventure.

Table 64.1.i. Some foods containing trace poisons

POISON	FOOD SOURCE

Cyanogens
  Linemarin,
  Laetrile
	Almonds, Lima beans, Tea,
	Cassava (manioc, tapioca),
	Bamboo shoots (immature),
	Various pips including Apple,
	Cherry, Peach and Apricot kernels

Dopa glycosides
  Vincine,
  Covincine
	Broad beans

Hypoglycaemics
  Hypoglycin A and B
  Anti-riboflavin
  Carnitine inhibitor
	Ackee (a tropical fruit)

Goitrogens (Iodine Antagonists)	Various Brassicas including Turnips, Broccoli, Brussels Sprouts, Cabbage, Kale and Cauliflower, Peanuts
Glucosinolates, Isothiocyanates	Mustard, Horseradish, Cabbage, Brussels sprouts, Spinach, Capers

Nitrates,
  Nitrites
  (form Nitrosamines)
	Cured meats, Bacon, Sausages,
	Salami

Oxalic acid	Almonds, Celery, Parsley, Spinach, Beetroot, Rhubarb, Cocoa, Various berries

Sapotoxins
  Solanine,
  Safrole
	Potatoes (if green), Aubergines

Continued /

Table 64.1.ii.

POISON	FOOD SOURCE
Trypsin inhibitors	Various legumes including Peanuts, Lima beans, Soya beans, Navy Beans, Peas, Sweet, Potatoes
Pyrrolizidine	Various Legumes
β–N-oxalyl-aminoalanine	Lathyrus (a poor-quality pulse)
Toxic amines Histamine	Various fish, Tuna, Mackerel, Eels (may also contain ciguatoxin)
Serotonin	Banana, Plantain (baking banana), Avocado, Pineapple, Strawberry, Tomatoes
Tyramine	Various cheeses, Yeast and Meat extracts, Salted Herring, Avocado

Xanthine alkaloids
  Caffeine,
  Theobromine,
  Theophylline
	Coffee, Tea, Cocoa, Cola

Phytic Acid	Various Grains including Wheat and Rye (includes gluten), Beans (in pod), Blackberries
Thujone	Wormwood (used to make Vermouth and Absinth)
Alcohol congeners	Alcoholic beverages

65

Dried Products, Herbs and Spices

Controlled drying or dehydration of certain foods is frequently carried out mainly as an aid to preserving the food. Such products generally have a much higher concentration of nutrients than their original levels. However, in many cases these products are not edible without first re-hydrating them. Following re-hydrating, cooking may also be necessary. For this reason, it is misleading to include such un-reconstituted foods in value tables. For example, dried pulses such as beans, peas and lentils are hardly ever eaten without first soaking and cooking them. Dried fruits, however, are occasionally eaten directly and are a rich source of nutrients including many vitamins. Also, dried milk is always reconstituted before use. Dried yeast, although used in the preparation of some foods, is best considered as a valuable natural supplement. Wheat germ, likewise, is a well-known very rich source of certain vitamins and essential amino acids. Wheat bran is also a somewhat unexpected source of certain vitamins, which also has the benefits of a high dietary fibre content. Honey is a concentrated sugar solution but contains only traces of other nutrients. The much-vaunted royal jelly is another rather esoteric bees' product, but is nevertheless an unusually good source of pantothenic acid. Pollen is also a rich source of the B-group vitamins. Yet, these foodstuffs can hardly be considered as regular foods as they are only available in supplementary form. Again, various oils, such as cod liver oil, contain virtually no water and are valuable sources of lipid-soluble vitamins. But they must be rated, for the most part, as supplements rather than as foodstuffs, although vegetable oils for cooking are increasing in popularity. Most raw foods, notably vegetables, contain higher concentrations of vitamins than they do after cooking or boiling (see Appendix A5). So, it is misleading to include the raw values in food tables unless the foods are normally eaten in the raw state, like salad vegetables for example. The vitamin content of brewer's yeast, wheat germ, and wheat bran, are given in Table 65.1. The high contents of many of the B-group vitamins are worth noting.

Herbs consist of the leaves, and occasionally other parts such as roots, bulbs and berries, of certain plants originally grown in temperate climates. Spices consist of certain aromatic seeds, fruit, flowers and bark of plants originally found in tropical climates. Herbs and spices have both culinary (nutritional) and medicinal (therapeutic) significance. The culinary value of herbs and spices resides more in their ability to flavour food than to any direct contribution of nutrients. That is not to say that they are devoid of vitamins and minerals. For example, parsley contains iron, comfrey contains calcium, phosphorous and potassium, alfalfa contains fat-soluble vitamins, garlic contains selenium, and so on. But in most diets these traces do not contribute significantly to the overall intake.

A large range of condiments and seasonings are derived from various fruit, berries and seeds, such as lemon juice, pepper, aromatic oils and vinegar, even alcoholic potions. The most common seasoning of all is salt, which is derived from the sea. Natural sea salt contains iodine and other trace minerals. Pickling in brine or vinegar is another way of preserving and preparing certain seasonal produce. Apart from disguising the taste of poor quality food, herbs and spices may act as preservatives. They may add flavour to bland starchy diets that are the staple food of Third World countries.

The medicinal value of herbs has been known for centuries and includes such cures as dock leaves for nettle stings and ginseng for impotence. Comfrey contains the healing agent allantoin, which helps to promote the formation of epithelial cells and hence speeds the healing of wounds, ulcers, and perhaps (because it also contains calcium and phosphorous) it is claimed, even broken bones. There is an analogy here between allantoin and ascorbic acid (vitamin C). Neither are produced to any extent in humans, yet enzymes are present in various other animals which enable these substances to be synthesised. While vitamin C is absolutely essential for good health, allantoin does not seem to be, hence it cannot be classified among the true vitamins. Nevertheless, since it has therapeutic properties, it could arguably be considered as one of the contingent nutrients. In any case, allantoin serves as a timely reminder that there are many more surprises in store for those who wish to explore and study the wonderful world of human nutrition.

Table 65.1. Comparison of some supplementary sources of vitamins
(all values per 100 grams)

VITAMIN	SOURCE		
	BAKER'S YEAST (dried)	WHEAT GERM	WHEAT BRAN
Water-Soluble			
Vitamin C (mg)	trace	nil	nil
The B-Group Vitamins			
Choline (mg)	32	150	74
Niacin (NE)	43	5.0	33
Pantothenic acid (mg)	11	2.4	2.4
Vitamin B_6 (mg)	2.0	1.0	1.4
Riboflavin (mg)	4.0	0.8	0.4
Thiamin (mg)	2.3 [a]	2.2	0.9
Folate (mg)	4.0	0.4	0.3
Biotin (mg)	0.2	negligible	trace
Vitamin B_{12} (mg)	trace [b]	negligible	nil
Fat-Soluble			
Vitamin E (TE)	trace	17.0	1.6
Vitamin A (RAE)	trace	nil	nil
Vitamin K (µg)	nil	trace	nil
Vitamin D (µg)	nil	trace	nil

a. Brewer's yeast contains a higher concentration of thiamin averaging
9.7 mg per 100 grams.

b. Sometimes the vitamin B_{12} content of dried yeast is increased (fortified).

A5

Loss of Vitamins

Stability and instability of the vitamins

Vitamin C

Least stable of the vitamins. Very easily destroyed by heat, oxygen, alkali, presence of copper in water or utensils. Lost by leaching. General losses during cooking amount to 40 – 60 percent. Losses during storage, even in a refrigerator, can be up to 100 percent.

Choline

Choline is heat-stable. Little of it is lost in most cooking processes. Choline remains at a constant level in dried foods over long periods. Choline ascorbate is highly stable.

Niacin

Very stable to most cooking processes. Lost by leaching. Typically, 10 – 25 percent is lost during cooking.

Pantothenic Acid

Relatively stable. Destroyed by heat, acid and alkali. Some losses by leaching. Typically, 10 – 20 percent is lost during cooking, but up to 40 percent may be lost on frying. Losses occur even during storage in a deep freezer.

Vitamin B_6

Very stable; pyridoxine being the most stable form. Lost by leaching. Typically, 25 – 50 percent is lost during cooking meat and vegetables.

Riboflavin

Stable on refrigeration. Destroyed by light and alkali, yielding lumiflavin. (Lumiflavin in turn destroys vitamin C.) Lost by leaching. Typically, 10 – 25 percent is lost during cooking.

Thiamine

Very unstable. Very easily destroyed by heat, alkali, some sulphur containing preservatives, and during food processing. Lost by leaching. Typically, 20 – 40 percent is lost during cooking. Up to 40 percent may be lost during cooking of vegetables. Up to 50 percent may be lost during cooking of meats.

Folate
Probably the least stable of the B-group vitamins. Destroyed by heat (and reheating) and light, particularly in the presence of riboflavin. Free folic acid is the unstable form of the vitamin. Folate is protected by vitamin C. Lost by leaching. Some losses during canning. Typically, 40 – 90 percent is lost during cooking of vegetables. However generally no loses occur during cooking of meats.

Biotin
Fairly stable. Lost by leaching. Typically, 10 – 30 percent is lost during cooking of meat and vegetables.

Vitamin B_{12}
Very stable. Destroyed by alkali and light. Protein protects vitamin B_{12}. Some lost by leaching. Typically, 10 – 25 percent is lost during cooking.

Vitamin E
Unstable. Destroyed by heat, alkali and during deep freezing. Lost during food processing. Up to 90 percent lost during bleaching of flour. Up to 80 percent lost on canning vegetables. Little loss during ordinary cooking but frying causes serious losses. Cooking of fats destroys some 70 – 90 percent of the vitamin E content. Up to 30 percent lost during the boiling of vegetables.

Vitamin A
Fairly stable. Destroyed by derivatives of polyunsaturated fatty acids (and Carotenoids) and oxygen. Protected by vitamin E. Little lost during ordinary cooking but decomposes on frying. Carotene levels may be reduced by 20 percent or more on drying of fruit or vegetables. Canning of green vegetables causes up to 20 percent loss, whereas canning of yellow or red vegetables may cause up to 35 percent loss.

Vitamin K

Stable. Destroyed by light. Some lost during food processing, and on deep freezing. Stable to most cooking methods. Probably up to 20 percent lost on average.

Vitamin D
Very stable, in fact provitamin D is activated by sunlight. Some losses during food processing, but very stable on smoking, drying, pasteurisation and sterilisation. Generally, stable to most cooking methods. Losses up to 25 percent have been reported for certain processes.

Modern food processing and canning methods conserve more of the vitamin content than in the past. Many foodstuffs are also fortified with added vitamins to compensate for deficiencies and losses.

Table A5.1.i. Vitamin losses during cooking and processing of various foods

FOOD GROUP	VITAMIN LOSSES (Average values)

MILK

Pasteurisation. Vitamin C, 30 percent; thiamine, 10 percent; and folate, 5 percent.

Boiling. Vitamin C, 50 percent; folate and vitamin E, 20 percent; vitamin B_6 and riboflavin, 10 percent; and vitamin B_{12}, 5 percent.

All methods including boiling, scrambling, frying and poaching. Folate, 10 – 35 percent; pantothenic acid, vitamin B_6 and riboflavin, 10 – 20 percent; and thiamine, 5 – 20 percent.

MEAT

Roasting, Frying, and Grilling. Vitamin C, niacin, pantothenic acid, vitamin B_6, riboflavin, thiamine, vitamin B_{12} and vitamin E, all 20 percent; biotin, 10 percent.

Stewing and Boiling. Thiamine, 60 percent; niacin and vitamin B_6, 50 percent; pantothenic acid, 40 percent; riboflavin and folate, 30 percent; vitamin C, vitamin B_{12} and vitamin E, 20 percent; and biotin, 10 percent.

All methods. All vitamin loses in meat are highly variable depending on the temperature and the duration of cooking.

All methods including poaching, frying, grilling and boiling. Thiamine, 10 – 30 percent; pantothenic acid, 20 percent; total folate, 0 – 20 percent (including up to 50 percent of the free folic acid); niacin, 10 – 20 percent; vitamin B_6 and riboflavin, 0 – 20 percent; biotin, 10 percent; and vitamin B_{12}, 0 – 10 percent.

Continued /

Table A5.1.ii.

FOOD GROUP	VITAMIN LOSSES (Average values)

GRAIN

Boiling. Total folate, 50 percent (including up to 90 percent of the free folic acid); niacin, pantothenic acid, vitamin B_6, riboflavin, thiamine and biotin, all 40 percent.

Baking. Total (and free) folate, 50 percent; pantothenic acid, vitamin B_6, and thiamine, 25 percent; riboflavin, 15 percent; and niacin, 5 percent.

VEGETABLES [1]

Boiling. Vitamin C, 40 – 70 percent; total folate, 20 – 50 percent (but up to 90 percent of the free folic acid); niacin, pantothenic acid, vitamin B_6 riboflavin, thiamine, and biotin, all 30 – 40 percent.

Freezing. Vitamin C, niacin, and riboflavin, 25 percent; thiamine, 20 percent; and vitamin A, 10 percent.

Canning. Thiamine, 65 percent; vitamin C and niacin, 50 percent; and vitamin A, 10 percent.

FRUIT

Freezing. Vitamin A, 40 percent; thiamine, 30 percent; vitamin C and riboflavin, 20 percent; and niacin, 15 percent.

Canning. Vitamin C and riboflavin, 55 percent; thiamine, 50 percent; niacin and vitamin A, 40 percent.

---

1. Vegetables here include pulses, root and leaf vegetables.

The irradiation of food also causes some vitamin losses.

A6

Experimental Depletion of Vitamins

In vitamin deficiency studies, onset times for symptoms to develop are highly variable and depend on the individual, the initial nutritional status, the age, sex, body size, percentage lipid, degree of activity, state of health, the balance of other nutrients in the diet, and many other variables. In many cases, controlled studies are extremely limited involving only a handful of volunteers. Total deprivation is rare. Minimal intake studies are more common as they are important in establishing daily intake requirements. The development of symptoms is often slow and involved and may proceed through several stages of increasing severity, not all of which can be followed experimentally. Furthermore, there is often a considerable time-lapse between the occurrence of some initial symptoms and the development of the final disease.

Table A6.1. summarises the average onset times for various vitamin deficiencies. For each value, it is assumed that total dietary deprivation of the vitamin and of no other nutrient is involved. The values given refer to normal healthy, mainly male adults, but are highly variable nevertheless. In the case of vitamin D, it should be recognised that the deficiency due to lack of vitamin D termed osteomalacia results in the resorption of calcium and phosphorous from the bones which may go on for a long time before deficiency is recognised. The condition should be distinguished from the much slower process called osteoporosis which is also characterised by a resorption of calcium and phosphorous from the bones which occurs in the elderly, particularly in women, but which is not directly due to a lack of vitamin D.

Table A6.1. Experimental depletion of vitamins

VITAMIN DEFICIENCY	ONSET TIME FOR MAIN SYMPTOMS TO DEVELOP (Days)
Vitamin C	150 – 180
Choline	20 – 40
Niacin	60, or longer [1]
Pantothenic Acid	70, or longer
Vitamin B_6	30, or longer
Riboflavin	100 – 130
Thiamine	150 – 200 [2]
Folate	120 – 150
Biotin	70, or longer [3]
Vitamin B_{12}	700 – 1,700
Vitamin E	500, or longer [4]
Vitamin A	300 – 1,000 [5]
Vitamin K	10 – 20 [6]
Vitamin D	300, or longer [7]

1. Tryptophan must also be absent because it can be converted to niacin in the body.

2. The rate of development of thiamine deficiency depends on the amount of carbohydrate in the diet.

3. Biotin deficiency possibly never occurs unless avidin is administered in combination with a low biotin diet.

4. There is a large store of vitamin E in the body and deficiency signs are difficult to induce, and may take years even on a high polyunsaturated fatty acid, low selenium, and low vitamin E regime. The onset time given above is therefore tentative.

5. Vitamin A and the carotenoids must be absent for deficiency to occur.

6. Vitamin K deficiency possibly never occurs in healthy individuals without administering antibiotics or warfarin.

7. Sunlight must also be absent for deficiency to occur. Also, the ratio of calcium to phosphorous and the level of calcium in the diet influence the onset time.

A7
Generic Descriptors for Vitamin Activity and Vitamers

Table A7.1.i. Generic descriptors for vitamin activity

GENERIC DESCRIPTOR	DEFINITION
Vitamin C	The term vitamin C is used as a generic descriptor for all compounds exhibiting qualitatively the biological (antiscorbutic) activity of L–ascorbic acid.
Niacin	The term niacin is used as a generic descriptor for pyridine–3–carboxylic acid and its derivatives exhibiting qualitatively the biological (antipellagric) activity of nicotinic acid.
Vitamin B_6	The term vitamin B_6 is used as a generic descriptor for all 3–hydroxy–2–methylpyridine derivatives exhibiting qualitatively the biological (antimicrocytic anemia, antiperipheral neuropathy, antidermatitis with cheilosis) activity of pyridoxine.
Folate	The term folate is used as a generic descriptor for compounds containing the pteroic acid nucleus exhibiting qualitatively the biological (hematopoietic) activity of tetrahydrofolic acid.
Vitamin B_{12}	The term vitamin B_{12} is used as a generic descriptor for all copper containing corrinoids exhibiting qualitatively the biological antipernicious anaemia) activity of cyanocobalamin.

Continued /

Table A7.1.ii.

GENERIC DESCRIPTOR	DEFINITION
Vitamin E	The term vitamin E is used as a generic descriptor for all tocopherols and tocotrienols exhibiting qualitatively the biological (antimyopathy, antiperipheral neuropathy, antimacrocytic anaemia, antisterility) activity of α-tocopherol.
Vitamin A [1,2]	The term vitamin A is used as a generic descriptor for all natural β-ionone derivatives, other than the provitamin A carotenoids, exhibiting qualitatively the biological (production and resynththesis of rhodopsin) activity of retinol.
Vitamin K	The term vitamin K is used as a generic descriptor for menadione and its derivatives exhibiting qualitatively the biological (formation of prothrombin) activity of phylloquinone.
Vitamin D [2]	The term vitamin D is used as a generic descriptor for all secosteroid derivatives exhibiting qualitatively the (antirachitic) biological activity of cholecalciferol.

1. The term retinoids may be used to describe both the natural and synthetic forms of retinol and its derivatives. And the terms retinol equivalent and retinol activity equivalent include the contribution of the provitamins to the total vitamin A activity.

2. The terms provitamin A and provitamin D are used to describe biologically inactive precursors that give rise to the corresponding active vitamins in the body.

Table A7.2. Natural vitamers

GENERIC DESCRIPTOR	NATURAL VITAMERS
Vitamin C	Ascorbic acid, Dehydroascorbic acid, Various salts of ascorbic acid
Choline	Choline, Betaine, CDP-Choline
Thiamine (B_1)	Thiamine, Thiamine pyrophosphate
Riboflavin (B_2)	Riboflavin, Flavin mononucleotide (FMN), Flavin adenine dinucleotide (FAD)
Niacin (B_3)	Niacinamide, Nicotinic acid
Pantothenic acid (B_5)	Pantothenic acid, Panthenol, Pantethine
Vitamin B_6	Pyridoxine, Pyridoxamine, Pyridoxal, Pyridoxal-5'-phosphate
Biotin (B_7)	D-Biotin, Dethiobiotin (DTB)
Folate (B_9)	Folic acid, Tetrahydrofolate, 5-Methyltetrahydrofolate, N5Formyltetrahydrofolic acid (Folinic acid)
Vitamin B_{12}	(Cyanocobalamin), Hydroxocobalamin, Methylcobalamin, Adenosylcobalamin or 5'-Deoxyadenosylcobalamin
Vitamin A	Retinol, Retinal and four Carotenoids: The Carotenes, alpha-Carotene, beta-Carotene, gamma-Carotene; and the Xanthophyll, beta-Cryptoxanthin
Vitamin D	Calcitriol, Ergocalciferol (D_2), Cholecalciferol (D_2)
Vitamin E	Tocopherols (d-alpha-, d-beta-, d-gamma- and d-delta-), Tocotrienols (alpha-, beta-, gamma- and delta-)
Vitamin K	Phylloquinone (K_1), Menaquinones (K_2)

A8

Vitamins as Coenzymes

Table A8.1.i. Vitamins as coenzymes

VITAMIN	COENZYME (OR ACTIVE) FORMS
Water–Soluble	
Vitamin C	None
The B-group Vitamins	
Choline	None
Niacin	Nicotine adenine dinucleotide (NAD) Nicotine adenine dinucleotide phosphate (NADP)
Pantothenic acid	Coenzyme A (CoA) and 4–Phosphopantetheine
Vitamin B_6	Pyridoxal phosphate / Pyridoxine phosphate
Riboflavin	Flavin mononucleotide (FMN) and Flavin adenine dinucleotide (FAD)
Thiamine	Thiamine pyrophosphate (TPP) Thiamine triphosphate (TTP)
Folate	Tetrahydrofolic acid (THFA), and derivatives [1]
Biotin	Biocytin
Vitamin B_{12}	Methylcobalamin and Adenosylcobalamin

1. Derivatives of THFA that act as coenzymes are listed in Chapter 54.

Continued /

Table A8.1.ii.

VITAMIN	COENZYME (OR ACTIVE) FORMS
Fat–Soluble	
Vitamin E [2]	None
Vitamin A	(11–cis–Retinal) [3]
Vitamin K [2, 4]	Vitamin K hydroquinone
Vitamin D	1,25–Dihydroxyvitamin D, and derivatives [5]

2. An electron carrier called ubiquinone (coenzyme Q, or CoQ), which is abundant in mitochondria, has some structural resemblance to both vitamin E and vitamin K.

3. The active forms of vitamin A are considered in Chapter 58.

4. During reactions the vitamin K coenzyme is converted to the 2,3–epoxide form.

5. The active forms of vitamin D are considered in Chapter 60.

A9

New Units for Older Vitamin Units

International Units

International Units (IU) were based on biological activity tests. However, because of improvements in the chemical measurement of vitamin compounds, these older units can now be replaced by milligram (mg) or microgram (µg) units as appropriate. Table A9.1 lists the appropriate conversion rates for some of these.

Equivalent Values

Vitamins are digested and absorbed at certain rates. In comparison, some provitamins are digested and absorbed at different rates than their corresponding vitamin and are converted to the active vitamin in the body after their uptake. The summation of the contributions of provitamins to the total biological activity of the vitamin requires a knowledge of the equivalent values of each component.

Imagine a vitamin has two provitamins, vitamer A and vitamer B, where 100 percent of vitamer A can be absorbed but only 25 percent of vitamer B can be absorbed. If they are both present in the diet in the same amounts, vitamer A will contribute four times more than vitamer B to the total biological activity. We can say that the value of vitamer B is only 0.25 biological equivalents, so the total intake will be 1.25 equivalents. Such equivalents have now been set for several provitamins as shown in Tables A9.2 to A9.5. Common equivalent values are summarised in Table A9.6.

Likewise, some vitamins are easier to absorb and utilise from certain sources in the diet than others and the differences can often be expressed in equivalent terms. So far, only a few vitamins have been assigned equivalents regarding defined sources or circumstances as shown in Table A9.5 and part of A9.6.

Metabolism

Even after absorption, provitamins must be converted to the active vitamin in the body. For example, provitamin D in the body still needs sunlight to become activated. Other provitamins need to be metabolised to the active form. The efficiency of these conversions may need to be taken into account when considering their equivalency.

In all cases, equivalents are most conveniently compared to the biological activity of a standard form of the vitamin, usually the most active or the most common or the most stable form, which is given a value of 1 equivalent unit. Some standards suggested for the purposes of summation are listed in Table A9.7.

Table A9.1. New vitamin units for older International Units *

VITAMIN	RELATIONSHIP BETWEEN OLD AND NEW UNITS
Vitamin C	1 IU vitamin C = 50 µg L–ascorbic acid [1]
Vitamin E	3 IU vitamin E = 2 mg vitamin E [2] or, more strictly, 2.013 mg d-α–tocopherol or 2.7 mg dl-α–tocopherol
Vitamin A	10 IU vitamin A = 3 µg vitamin A [3] or, more strictly, 3 µg all-*trans*-retinol
Vitamin D	40 IU vitamin D = 1 µg vitamin D [4] or, more strictly, 1 µg cholecalciferol (vitamin D_3) or 1 µg ergocalciferol (vitamin D_2)

* From July 2019, International Units will no longer be used for vitamins E, A and D.

1. International Units are no longer used for vitamin C.

2. 1.49 IU vitamin E = 1 mg α–tocopherol equivalent by definition. So, 1 IU vitamin E = 0.67 mg α–tocopherol equivalent (TE).

3. 1 IU vitamin A = 0.3 µg retinol activity equivalents (RAE).

4. 1 IU vitamin D = 0.025 mg cholecalciferol or ergocalciferol.

Table A9.2. Tocopherol equivalents (TE) associated with vitamers of vitamin E in the human

COMPOUND	TE (milligrams)
1 mg α–Tocopherol	1.00
1 mg β–Tocopherol	0.50
1 mg γ–Tocopherol	0.10
1 mg δ–Tocopherol	0.01
1 mg α–Tocotrienol	0.30
1 mg β–Tocotrienol	0.05
1 mg γ–Tocotrienol	----
1 mg δ–Tocotrienol	----

Table A9.3. Retinol activity equivalents (RAE)* associated with vitamers of vitamin A in the human

COMPOUND	RAE (micrograms)
1 µg all-*trans*-Retinol	1
1 µg all-*trans*-β-Carotene (from oil)	0.5
1 µg all-*trans*-β-Carotene (from food)	0.083
1 µg α-Carotene	0.042
1 µg γ-Carotene	0.042
1 µg β-Zeacarotene	0.042
1 µg β-Cryptoxanthin	0.042

* To be distinguished from retinol equivalents (RE) which are inaccurate. Since 2001, RE has been replaced by RAE.

Table A9.4. Niacin Equivalents (NE) associated with vitamers of niacin in the human

COMPOUND	NE (milligrams)
1 mg of Nicotinamide	1
1 mg of Nicotinic acid	1
1 mg Tryptophan	0.0167

Table A9.5. Dietary Folate Equivalents (DFE) depend on sources and circumstances *

COMPOUND	DFE (micrograms)
1 µg natural folates derived from unfortified food	1.00
1 µg folic acid derived from fortified food or supplements taken with food	1.67
1 µg folic acid derived from supplements taken on an empty stomach	2.00

* To calculate the DFE of a fortified food, it is necessary to know the micrograms of natural folate and synthetic folic acid present.

The Total DFE is given as 1 x µg natural folates plus 1.67 x µg synthetic folic acid.

Table A9.6. Common equivalent values

Tocopherol Equivalent (TE)

1 mg TE	= 1 mg α-Tocopherol
1 mg TE	= 2 mg β–Tocopherol
1 mg TE	= 3.3 mg α–Tocotrienol
1 mg TE	= 10 mg γ–Tocopherol
1 mg TE	= 20 mg β–Tocotrienol
1 mg TE	= 100 mg δ–Tocopherol

Retinal Activity Equivalent (RAE)

1 μg RAE	= 1 μg Retinol (specifically all-*trans*-retinol)
1 μg RAE	= 2 μg all-*trans*-β-carotene derived from oil
1 μg RAE	= 12 μg all-*trans*-β-carotene derived from food
1 μg RAE	= 24 μg other provitamin A carotenoids *

Niacin Equivalent (NE)

1 mg NE	= 1 mg of Nicotinamide
1 mg NE	= 1 mg of Nicotinic acid
1 mg NE	= 60 mg of Tryptophan

Dietary Folate Equivalent (DFE)

1 μg DFE	= 1 μg Folate derived from unfortified food
1 μg DFE	= 0.6 μg Folic acid derived from fortified food or supplements taken with food
1 μg DFE	= 0.5 μg Folic acid derived from supplements taken on an empty stomach

---

* Including *α-Carotene, γ-Carotene, β-*Zeacarotene and *β-Cryptoxanthin.*

Table A9.7. Other possible reference compounds to establish equivalent values

VITAMIN	REFERENCE COMPOUND
Vitamin C	L-Ascorbic acid equivalent
Choline	Choline equivalent
Niacin	Nicotinamide equivalent
Pantothenic acid	Pantothenic acid equivalent
Vitamin B_6	Pyridoxine equivalent
Riboflavin	Riboflavin equivalent
Thiamine	Thiamine equivalent
Folate	Folic acid equivalent
Biotin	Biotin equivalent
Vitamin B_{12}	Cyanocobalamin equivalent
Vitamin E	RRR-α-Tocopherol equivalent
Vitamin A	all-*trans*-Retinol equivalent
Vitamin K	Phylloquinone equivalent
Vitamin D	Cholecalciferol or Ergocalciferol equivalent

A10

Common Toxicity and Deficiency Symptoms of the Vitamins

Table A10.1.i. Common toxicity and deficiency symptoms of vitamins

NUTRIENT	TOXICITY	DEFICIENCY
Water–soluble vitamins		
Vitamin C	Possible kidney stones.	Scurvy.
The B-group Vitamins		
Choline	Lowered blood pressure. Excessive sweating. Salivation. A fishy body odor. Gastrointestinal disturbances.	Fatigue. Nerve damage. Muscle damage. Fatty liver. Cognitive impairment. Mood changes.
Niacin	Tingling. Possibly temporary flushing of the skin. Headaches. Liver disorders. B-group vitamin imbalance.	Pellagra. Enzyme disorders.
Riboflavin	Harmless yellow colouration of urine. B-group vitamin imbalance.	Cheilosis. Enzyme disorders.
Vitamin B$_6$	High doses may cause tingling sensations. Numbness. Polyneuropathy. B-group vitamin imbalance.	Infantile convulsions. Enzyme disorders. Psychic disturbances.

Continued /

Table A10.1.ii.

NUTRIENT	TOXICITY	DEFICIENCY

Water–soluble vitamins, continued

NUTRIENT	TOXICITY	DEFICIENCY
Pantothenic acid	B-group vitamin imbalance.	Vague symptoms. Cramps. Fatigue. insomnia. Nausea. Poor coordination. Enzyme disorders.
Thiamine	Beriberi. Polyneuritis. Rare allergic reactions.	B-group vitamin imbalance. Enzyme disorders.
Biotin	Fatigue. Depression.	B-group vitamin imbalance. Nausea. Dermatitis. Muscle pains. Enzyme disorders.
Folate	May mask vitamin B_{12} deficiency.	B-group vitamin imbalance. Megaloblastic (macrocytic) anaemia. Bowel disturbances. Diarrhoea (Sprue).
Vitamin B_{12}	B-group vitamin imbalance is unlikely. Very rare allergic reactions.	Pernicious anaemia. Peripheral neuropathy. Fatigue. Secondary folate deficiency. Methylmalonic acid buildup.

Continued /

Table A10.1.iii.

NUTRIENT	TOXICITY	DEFICIENCY

Lipid–soluble vitamins

NUTRIENT	TOXICITY	DEFICIENCY
Vitamin E	Non–specific symptoms. Possibly blurred vision. Headaches. Palpitations	Anaemia in neonatal infants. Not known in adults. Muscle weakness.
Vitamin A	Liver enlargement. Nausea, Headaches, Pigmentation of face. Peeling of skin. Hair loss. Anorexia.	Night Blindness, Severe growth retardation. Bone abnormalities in children. Keratinization of various soft tissues including the eyes (Xerothalmia). Glandular and lung disorders. Sterility. Eventual permanent blindness.
Vitamin K	Kernictus. Haemolytic anaemia (Jaundice). Vomiting. Liver damage. Kidney damage.	Haemorrhagic disease in infants. Defective blood clotting in adults.
Vitamin D	Hypercalcemia. Abnormal deposition of calcium. Kidney damage. Vomiting. Diarrhoea, Weight loss.	Rickets in children. Osteomalacia in adults.

Bibliography

General Reading

Bryce-Smyth, D. and Hodgkinson, L. (1986). The zinc solution, Century Arrow.

Burkitt, D. (1982). Don't forget the fibre in your diet, Third edition, Martin Dunitz.

Candlish, J. (1981). Metabolic water and the camel's hump—a textbook survey, *Biochemical Education* 9(3) 1981 96-97.

Cathie, K. (1976). The complete calorie counter, Pan Books.

Cathie, K. (1978). The complete carbohydrate counter, Pan Books.

Chaitow, L. (1985). Amino acids in therapy, Thorsons.

Forbes, A. (1990). Healthy eating: cooking with vitamins and minerals, Penguin Books.

Graham, J. and Odent, M. (1986). The Z factor, Thorsons.

Lewis, A. (1983). Selenium, Revised Expanded Edition Thorsons.

Mervyn, L. (1981). The B vitamins, Thorsons.

Mervyn, L. (1981). Vitamin C, Thorsons.

Mervyn, L. (1984). Vitamin E, Revised Edition, Nature's Way Series, Thorsons.

Mervyn, L. (1984). Vitamins A, D, K, Nature's Series, Thorsons.

Sherman, A. (1984). The sodium counter, Arlington Books.

Thomas, J. (1985). The fat counter, Pan Books.

Trimmer, E. (1987). The magic of magnesium, Thorsons.

Tudge, C. (1985). The food connection, BBC Publication.

Wright, M. (1984). The salt counter, Pan Books.

Encyclopedias and Dictionaries

Adrian, J., Legrand, G and Frange, R. (1988). Dictionary of food and nutrition. Translator, B. Weitz. Translation Editors, E. Rolfe, I. Morton and L. Mabbit Ellis Horwood.

Black's agricultural dictionary, (1981). Edited by D. B. Dalal-Clayton Adam and Charles Black, Black Publishers Ltd.

Butterworth' s dictionary of nutrition and food technology, (1982). Edited by A. E. Bender, Butterworths.

Campion, K. (1986). Vegetarian encyclopedia, Century paperbacks.

Fischer, R. B. (1986). A dictionary of diets, slimming and nutrition, Paladin.

Illustrated Stedman's medical dictionary, (1982). 24th Edition, Williams and

Wilkins.
Kirschmann, J. D. (1979). Nutrition almanac, Revised Fourth Edition, McGraw-Hill.
Mayes, A. (1986). The dictionary of nutritional health: guide to the relation between diet and health, Thorsons.
McGraw-Hill Encyclopedia of food, agriculture and nutrition, (1977). Edited by D. N. Lapedes, McGraw-Hill.
Mervyn, L. (1986). Thorsons' complete guide to vitamins and minerals, Thorsons.
Scott, T. and Brewer, M. (1983). Concise encyclopedia of biochemistry, Walter de Gruyter.
Stenesh, J. (1975). Dictionary of biochemistry, John Wiley and Sons.
The encyclopedia of the biological sciences, (1983). Edited by P. Gray, Second Edition Van Nostrand.
Van Nostrand's scientific encyclopedia, (1983). Edited by D. M. Considine and G. D. Considine, Sixth Edition, Van Nostrand.
W. B. Saunders' atomic energy encyclopedia in the life sciences, (1964). Edited by C. Shilling, W. B. Saunders.
Yudkin, J. (1985). The penguin encyclopedia of nutrition, Penguin Books.

Textbooks

Bell, G. H., Davison, J. N. and Emslie-Smyth, D. (1972). Textbook of physiology and biochemistry, Eight Edition, Churchill Livingstone.
Bohinski, H. C. (l979). Modern concepts in biochemistry, Third Edition, Allyn and Bacon.
Bowman, C. and Rand, M. J. (1980). Textbook of pharmacology, Second Edition, Blackwell Scientific Publications.
Burton, B. T. (1976). Human nutrition, Third Edition, McGraw-Hill.
Davidson and Passmore's human nutrition and dietetics, (1986). 8th Edition, Edited by R. Passmore and M. A. Eastwood, Churchill Livingstone.
Ganong, F. (1987). Review of medical physiology, Thirteenth Edition, Lange Medical Publications.
Gibney, M. J. (1986). Nutrition, diet and health, Cambridge University Press.
Goodman and Gillman's the pharmacological basis of therapeutics, (1985). Seventh Edition, Edited by A. G. Gilman, L. S. Goodman, T. W. Rall and F. Murad, Macmillan.
Green, J. H. (1980). An introduction to human physiology, Fourth (SI) Revised Edition, Oxford University Press.
Gurr, M. I. (l984). Role of fats in food and nutrition, Elsevier Applied Science Publishers.

Gurr, M. I. and James, A. T. (1975). Lipid biochemistry, Second Edition, Chapman and Hall.

Guyton, A. C. (2006). Textbook of medical physiology, Eleventh Edition, W. B. Saunders.

Katzung, B. G. (Editor) (1984). Basic clinical pharmacology, 2nd Edition, Lange Medical Publications.

Lehninger, A. L. (1982). Principles of Biochemistry, Worth Publishers Inc.

Lloyde, L. E., McDonald, B. E. and Crampton, E. W. (1978). Fundamentals of nutrition, Second Edition, W. H. Freeman and Co.

McDonald, P., Edwards, R. A. and Greenhalgh, J. F. D. (1988). Animal nutrition, Longman, Scientific and Technical.

Metzler, D. E. (1977). Biochemistry: the chemical reactions of living cells, Academic Press.

Murray, R. K., Granner, D. K., Mayes, P. A. and Rodwell, V. W. (1990). Harper's biochemistry, Twenty-second Edition, Lange Medical Books.

Ottaway, J. H. and Apps, D. K. (1984). Biochemistry, Fourth Edition, Baillière Tyndall.

Peterson, C. R. (1983). Essentials of human biochemistry, Pitman Books.

Smith, E. L., Hill, R. L., Lehman, I. R., Lefkowitz, R. J., Handler, P. and White, A. (1983). Principles of biochemistry: mammalian biochemistry, Seventh Edition McGraw-Hill.

Taylor, T. G. (1978). Principles of human nutrition, The Institute of Biology Series No 94, Edward Arnold.

Vander, A. J., Sherman, J. H. and Luciane, D. S. (1984). Human physiology: the mechanism of body function, Fourth Edition, McGraw-Hill.

Wills, E. D. (1985). Biochemical basis of medicine, John Wright and Sons.

Reference Works

Assmann, G. (1982). Lipid metabolism and atherosclerosis, F. K. Schattauer Verlag.

Bender, A. E. and Bender, D. A. (1986). Food tables, Oxford University Press.

Biochemical nomenclature and related documents, (1978). International Union of Biochemistry, as reprinted for the Biochemical Society by Spottiswoode Ballantyne Press.

Biological handbooks (new series) Vol II: Human health and disease, (1977). Edited by P. L. Altman and D. Dittmer Katz, Fed. Amer. Soc. Exp. Biol., Bethesda, Maryland.

Biological handbooks: blood and other body fluids (1961). Edited by P. L. Altman and D. S. Dittmer, Fed. Amer. Soc. Exp. Biol., Bethesda, Maryland.

Biological handbooks: metabolism, (1968). Edited by P. L. Altman and D.

S. Dittmer, Fed. Amer. Soc. Exp. Biol., Bethesda, Maryland.

CRC handbook of biochemistry: selected data for molecular biology, (1970). 2nd Edition, Edited by H. A. Sober, CRC Press.

CRC handbook of chemistry and physics, (1981). 62nd Edition, Edited by R. C. Weast and M. J. Astle, CRC Press.

CRC handbook of eicosanoids: prostaglandins and related lipids, Vol I (Part A): Biochemical aspects (1987). Edited by A. L. Willis, CRC Press.

CRC handbook series. Nutrition and food: Section E, nutritional disorders, Vol I. Effects of nutrient excesses and toxicities in animals and man, (1977). Edited by M. Rechcigl, Jr., CRC Press.

Food and agriculture organisation: energy yielding components of food and computation of caloric values. (1947). F.A.O. Nutrition Division.

Food, nutrition and climate (1982). Edited by K. Blaxter and L. Fowden, Applied Science Publishers.

Geigy Scientific Tables: Eight revised and enlarged edition, Edited by C. Lentner, Ciba-Geigy.

Handbook of vitamins: nutritional, biochemical and clinical aspects (1984). Edited by L. J. Machlin, Marcel Dekker.

Nutrient interactions, (1988). Edited by C. E. Bodwell and J. W. Erdman, Jr., Marcel Dekker.

Osborne, D. R. and Voogt, P. (1978). The analysis of nutrients in foods, Academic Press.

Paul, A. A. and Southgate, D. A. T. (1978). McCance and Widdowson's the composition of foods, Fourth Edition, H. M. Stationary Office London.

Paul, A. A., Southgate, D. A. T., and Russell, J. (1980). First supplement to McCance and Widdowson's the composition of foods, H. M. Stationary Office London.

Reeds, P. J., (2000). "Dispensable and indispensable amino acids for humans", *American Society for Nutritional Sciences, Supplement.* 1835S–1840S.

Recommended dietary allowances (1989). Tenth Edition, Food and Nutrition Board, National Academy of Sciences - National Research Council, US.

Requirements of vitamin A, iron, folate and vitamin B12 (1988). Report of joint FAO/WHO expert consultation. Food and Agriculture Organisation of the United Nations, Rome.

Shamberger, R. J. (1983). Biochemistry of the elements: Vol 2. Biochemistry of selenium, Plenum Press.

Trace elements in human and animal nutrition: Vol 2 (1986). Fifth Edition, Edited by W. Mertz, Orlando, Academic Press.

Van Dorp, P. A. (1973). Essential fatty acids and prostaglandins: Vol 2. Butterworths.

World Health Organisation: handbook on human nutritional requirements

(1974). Monograph Series No. 61, WHO in collaboration with the Food and Agriculture Organisation of the United Nations.

Web Sources

Dietary Reference Intakes, (1997 – 2011). National Academies Press.

Dietary Reference Intakes for Calcium, Phosphorous, Magnesium, Vitamin D, and Fluoride (1997);

Dietary Reference Intakes for Thiamin, Riboflavin, Niacin, Vitamin B6, Folate, Vitamin B12, Pantothenic Acid, Biotin, and Choline (1998);

Dietary Reference Intakes for Vitamin C, Vitamin E, Selenium, and Carotenoids (2000);

Dietary Reference Intakes for Vitamin A, Vitamin K, Arsenic, Boron, Chromium, Copper, Iodine, Iron, Manganese, Molybdenum, Nickel, Silicon, Vanadium, and Zinc (2001);

Dietary Reference Intakes for Energy, Carbohydrate, Fiber, Fat, Fatty Acids, Cholesterol, Protein, and Amino Acids (2002/2005);

Dietary Reference Intakes for Calcium and Vitamin D (2011);

Note: These reports may be accessed via: *www.nap.edu* .

Dietary Reference Intakes (DRIs): Estimated Average Requirements. Food and Nutrition Board, Institute of Medicine, National Academies. Life Stage. Group. *https://fnic.nal.usda.gov/sites/fnic.nal.usda.gov/files/uploads/recommended_ intakes_individuals.pdf* [modified: 16 December 2015].

United States Department of Agriculture, National Agricultural Library (USDA, NAL), DRI Tables and Application Reports, *https://fnic.nal.usda.gov/dietary-guidance/dietary-reference-intakes* [modified: 30 April 2016].

https://fnic.nal.usda.gov/dietary-guidance/dietary-reference-intakes/ dri-tables-and-application-reports [retrieved: 28 September 2016].

Dietary Reference Intakes (DRIs) are developed and published by the Institute of Medicine (IOM). The DRIs represent the most current scientific knowledge on nutrient needs of healthy populations.

Dietary Reference Intakes for Energy, Carbohydrate, Fiber, Fat, Fatty Acids, Cholesterol, Protein, and Amino Acids (Macronutrients), (2005). National Academies Press. *http://www.nap.edu/catalog/10490/ dietary-reference-intakes-for-energy-carbohydrate-fiber-fat-fatty-acids-cholesterol-protein-and-amino-acids-macronutrients* [modified: 7 April 2016].

Linus Pauling Institute, Micronutrient Information Center. Oregon State University. Choline, *http://lpi.oregonstate.edu/mic/other-nutrients/choline* [retrieved: 29 April 2016].

Linus Pauling Institute, Micronutrient Information Center. Oregon State University. Essential Fatty Acids, *http://lpi.oregonstate.edu/mic/other-nutrients/essential-fatty-acids* [retrieved: 28 September 2016].

The Linus Pauling Institute is a valuable authoritative source of information on the nutrients.

Payne, P.R., (1971). Reference protein patterns, 1–8, *ftp://ftp.fao.org/docrep/fao/meeting/009/ae906e/ae906e25.pdf* [modified: 12 October 2016].

Supplements-And-Health.com. (2016). Lesser Known Facts About Tryptophan Side Effects. *http://www.supplements-and-health.com/tryptophan-side-effects.html* [retrieved: 21 October 2016].

University of Maryland Medical Centre. (2016). Phenylalanine, *http://umm.edu/health/medical/altmed/supplement/phenylalanine* [retrieved: 17 October 2016].

US Department of Agriculture, National Agricultural Library. (2016). DRI Nutrient Reports. https://fnic.nal.usda.gov/dietary-guidance/dietary-reference-intakes/dri-nutrient-reports [retrieved, 18 October 2016].

Wikipedia. (2016). "Essential amino acid", *https://en.wikipedia.org/wiki/Essential_amino_acid* [modified: 11 October 2016].

About the Author

Richard Rydon

Richard Rydon is an award-winning science fiction novelist. His three books in the Luper Series, The Oortian Summer (2007), The Omega Wave (2008) and The Palomar Paradox: A SETI Mystery (2011), have been given excellent reviews.

Richard's second novel, The Omega Wave, was selected as one of the finalists in the Science Fiction Category of the Reader Views Literary Awards and was awarded an Honorary Mention (Third Place) in the Reviewers Choice Awards in 2009.

His third novel, The Palomar Paradox, won the Bronze/3rd Place award in the Romance Category of the Feathered Quill Book Awards in 2014.

Richard is an honours science graduate. He has also obtained numerous certificates and diplomas in Psychology, Counselling, Theology, and a Diplôme de Cuisine Française. He is a prolific writer and has published over 300 papers, articles and poems, in scientific journals, magazines and local papers to date.

He has also published a second edition of his anthology of poetry, titled A Golden Fuchsia-Laden Girl (2011), containing 100 poems.

About the Science Fiction Novels in the Luper Series

The Oortian Summer

'The Oortian Summer' is a romantic science fiction adventure involving co-worker relationships in an astronomical observatory as two massive comets approach the Earth. The unusual twist in the story involves a perilous attempt, proposed by Luper, the lead character, to bring the comets even closer to Earth to prevent a catastrophic geomagnetic flip.

The Omega Wave

'The Omega Wave' is a gothic science fiction novel. Aided and abetted by Quade their boss, Luper and Frieda progress secretly and meticulously, to develop biological computers called neurospheres. Working in the shadow of a rogue American Embassy, they first conceal but later reveal what they have seen and done.

The Palomar Paradox: A SETI Mystery

'The Palomar Paradox' sees Luper back in an astronomical observatory searching for signs of extraterrestrial intelligence. He finds himself working with Leila, a young girl recovering from leukaemia, and Karina, an experienced astronomer, among others. As their research continues, unusual signals are picked up by their radio telescope. The signals are explained, one by one, until … !

About Richard Rydon's Poetry

A Golden Fuchsia-Laden Girl

'A Golden Fuchsia-Laden Girl' is an anthology of one hundred poems of whimsy, innocence and longing, by Richard Rydon, written and revised between 1957 and 2011. Twenty poems have been added in this second edition.

About Richard Rydon's Non-Fiction Books

Matter, Energy and Mentality: Exploring Metaphysical Reality

His non-fiction book, 'Matter, Energy and Mentality: Exploring Metaphysical Reality', was published in 2012. 'Matter, Energy and Mentality' is a book of speculative non-fiction. It covers the relationships between Matter, Energy and Mentality, using Energy Redistribution (Unnecessary Action) as a common feature in the Universe.

Profiles of the Nutrients

'Profiles of the Nutrients — 1. Carbohydrate, Lipid, and Protein' published in 2016, is the first book in a series about the nutrients which are essential for human life.

The other books in the series are titled as follows:
'Profiles of the Nutrients — 2. Minerals and Trace Elements'.

'Profiles of the Nutrients — 3. Water-Soluble and Fat-Soluble Vitamins'.